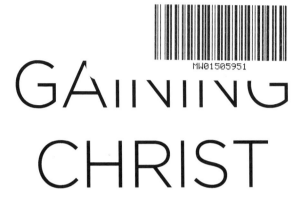

GAINING
CHRIST

A Weight Loss Devotional

KRISTY LOEWEN

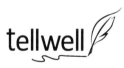

Tellwell Talent
www.tellwell.ca

ISBN
978-0-2288-3551-6 (Paperback)
978-0-2288-3552-3 (eBook)

TABLE OF CONTENTS

DEDICATION

To my Heavenly Father: being able to share your thoughts through my experiences is reason enough for it all to have happened.

To my husband: you have always put up with my shenanigans. I wouldn't be here without you.

To my two toddlers: I can honestly say that this book would not have been as insightful without you in my life. You cannot buy the exprcience having kids gives you. The fact that I have any hair left is proof there is a God.

To my family and friends who have supported me in this dream.

To everyone who has ever had issues with their weight. I had no idea what you were going through until I experienced it for myself in recent years. It has been an eye-opening and empathetic journey thus far. Don't lose hope! I haven't.

To anyone who has ever tried to help someone else lose weight, please stop trying to fix us. Instead, offer prayer without being asked to do so. Offer your support without judgment when asked for it. And please try to see the circumstances that led us to this point, rather than our inability to get around them. God has an unfailing plan, and our journey through this is part of it.

FOREWORD

There is an irrevocable connection between our bodies and our souls—the state of one affects the state of the other. There are two ditches that we must avoid: one is focusing on the body to the neglect of the soul. Some people are fanatical about physical health but their souls are shrivelling; therefore, they struggle with finding peace and purpose. Those in the other ditch focus on their souls to the neglect of their bodies. This group seeks to nourish their souls through regular spiritual practices but their bodies are fighting against them; their souls are attempting to thrive in a toxic physical environment. We need to find the balance between these two ditches and strive for holistic health—physical *and* spiritual.

The Bible says in Galatians 5:23 that a fruit of the Spirit is self-control, and real self-control cannot be compartmentalized. If we have a difficult time saying no to a snack, then we will have a difficult time saying no to a sin. Self-control is a fruit of the Spirit that gets exercised through our choices.

We must *choose* to be holy.

We must *choose* to be healthy.

This forty-day devotional is a helpful tool for anyone wanting to be holistically healthy. Kristy doesn't write from an ivory tower of academia but rather from the front lines. She offers helpful insights from the real world. The content is biblical and authentic, which is what makes it helpful.

As Kristy states in her book, "Your purpose is right now. Your purpose is to submit, learn, and love. God's main purpose for your life is to further His kingdom, so where you are right now is all part of His plan. Look for it. Pray about it. Submit to the plan. Resist the devil and his foolish schemes. And come near to God."

For God's glory and our good,

John Schaffner

INTRODUCTION

This book is the culmination of twenty years of struggles and successes. I am constantly reminded that there is a reason God only shows us one or two steps ahead of where we are. If you had told me He was ultimately leading me to write Christian based nutrition books, I would've fought it.

I had wanted to be a pharmacist since I was in grade six. When I didn't get into the program in my second year of university, I was crushed. I planned to spend another year trying to improve my grades so I could apply again. God had other plans. The day before I had to register for classes, my kitten (who never sat still for more than two seconds) fell asleep in my arms as I did my devotionals that morning. Obviously, I couldn't move, so instead I just prayed. God brought nutrition to mind. It was a revelation but also just a *Why didn't I think of that?* moment. I have always loved nutrition, and it worked perfectly with my love of fitness. I could see my future laid out before me in an instant.

The next day I talked to about five different people at the university trying to figure out how to make something in the nutrition field happen. I knew it would be a long shot because I was late in all aspects. Let's just say that a process that should've taken months took me two hours. Every person I spoke to did what they needed to do right in front of me. I was amazed.

Fast forward three years to the end of university and onto conducting nutrition research. I loved my job. The professors who I worked with were amazing. They kept trying to convince me to do my master's degree with them, but I refused every time because I hated writing. I took science so I didn't have to write.

Fast forward another eight years. I wrote a sixteen-week manual for a healthy living program for seniors. Realizing writing wasn't so bad when I could break it up into chunks, I started to gain this picture of writing a nutrition-based Bible study. I knew I could break it up into chunks and it would be manageable. When I started to realize that this was what God was calling me to, I accepted the challenge. God confirmed this dream when a well-known publishing company called me out of the blue, asking me if my book was done yet. WHAT?! The caller ID confirmed that it was not a joke. God was just telling me it was time to start writing.

The rest of it happened very gradually. It has been another five years since that realization. In that time, I outlined about five different books, gained some weight due to unforeseen life events, had two babies and suffered a broken ankle when the first was seven months old and I was pregnant with the next one. I also took an eating psychology course while on maternity leave with the second. Am I crazy? No. Fitness and nutrition have always been the things I love, and they have kept me sane through the crazy of raising kids. After that I knew what was meant to happen next. This book.

It started off being a thirty-day devotional but it just never sat well. It was a great idea but something about it was wrong. Then God brought the forty-day desert to mind. So many trials in the Bible were associated with forty days, so it became a forty-day devotional. I slowly got an outline together but I could never figure out a name. I do my best thinking in the car or the bathtub and, finally, while I was driving some tired kids home from the park, the name came to me. The focus is Christ. Add a cute little pun and the rest is history.

I have not struggled with weight-related issues for most of my life, but when you put together some crazy life events, two kids, and a plan from God, the weight came on. Don't get me wrong, I don't like it. I am certain, though, that this book would not be effective without it. I am a firm believer that you cannot truly understand someone until you have gone through something similar yourself. I think that's why I've been through as much as I have. I know that my first-hand knowledge will make my writing more powerful and relatable.

I want you to know that your struggles are my struggles. The best part is that both of our struggles are in the ever-powerful hands of God. Nothing is impossible for God.

You are not a disappointment.

Read that again: You are not a disappointment.

God will never love you any more or any less than He does right now. When you feel you have nothing else to be thankful for, be thankful for that.

HOW TO USE THIS BOOK

This book is meant to encourage, and it can be read in any way that works best for you. I meant it to be completed in forty days but you could read it however you like. Maybe you know you have a longer journey ahead of you and you want to spread it out more. You could read one entry a week and have it last forty weeks. You could re-read that one day for seven days. That's your choice. God will reveal insights to you if you are open to it. If you find one day really triggers something for you, then maybe meditate on it for a few days before moving on. There are no rules and no set time length. I know many people don't like to be told what to do (me included), so I'd like you to follow your heart. Might sound kind of lame, but it is true. If you're open to it, God will make you aware.

In this book, when it comes to nutrition advice, there is very little. Yes, that is what I do for a living, and if you are interested in that, you can check out my website for more information at www.kristyloewen.com. This book is to encourage you in whatever method you are choosing to lose weight. Let me try to affirm you in your current choices. How many people are there in the world? Well, that's how many "ideal" diets there are. You need to find what works for you. That's how I run my business. In terms of exercise? Just remember that you cannot eat your way to bigger muscles. You exercise for that. How you eat may encourage that process, but if you do not exercise your muscles, you will not build any. Also, if you hate the kind of exercise you are doing, try changing it up. You will get much further in your exercise journey if you do not hate what you are doing. Mentally, it makes a big difference if you love what you are doing, rather than making it feel like punishment.

What if, instead of committing to our health and wellness plan, we commit to God himself? What if our commitment for the next forty devotionals was to write out all of our health and wellness goals, commit them to God, and then commit to devotion to God? Devotion to the One who created our very being. The One who knows us better than we know ourselves, what and who we were meant to be. In the absolute very least, we would gain what we should all desire first and foremost: a better relationship with our Creator. In the end, if that is all we gained, that is so much more than losing weight anyway, isn't it? But I would venture to guess that God wants us to be healthy as much as we do, so I think some change or shift may happen.

Just know that I am praying for you often. I pray for those God is bringing to this book. I pray that it will genuinely hit you right in the heart, and that it will help transform your mind and body along with it.

> *Forget about self-confidence; it's useless. Cultivate God-confidence. No test or temptation that comes your way is beyond the course of what others have had to face. All you need to remember is that God will never let you down; He'll never let you be pushed past your limit; He'll always be there to help you come through it.*
>
> —*1 Corinthians 10:12-13 The Message*

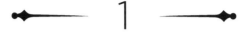

ROCK BOTTOM

Welcome to this forty-day devotional. I am going to make an assumption right off the top that many of you reading this are at rock bottom. At the very least, you're frustrated with your weight situation.

You have come to the right place.

All I ask is that you open your heart to God and what He has to say to you through this book. Let's get to it!

I've been thinking about the saying "rock bottom" lately. As someone who has been through some hard times, rock bottom is not a place I would like to go again. When I had depression, at the very worst times, I realized I had lost who I was completely. I lost my personality. I lost logic. I lost sleep. I lost the things I loved, like fitness, the outdoors, and friends. It was only when I hit rock bottom, however, that I realized I was finally low enough to find my foundation. Rock bottom is as low as it gets. But rock itself is solid. I may have broken down what I thought to be every important part of me, but I was really just digging deeper to find what I built my life on: Christ.

Christ was my rock bottom. He was the only thing I never lost on the way down. He was always just one thought away. He was the one who encouraged me to tell someone. He was the one who helped me bring it to the light. He was the one whose name I could utter and feel some relief. And when I got strong enough, I moved from asking Him to fight my fights, to helping Him.

There were three very clear stages to my depression. When I was at my lowest, all I could do was say "Jesus." When I started rebuilding on my rock bottom, I moved to saying, "Jesus, please fight this for me." And finally, when my foundation and walls were firm, Jesus handed me the sword and said, "It's your turn to join me. Let's fight this together."

Your weight loss journey may feel the same. If you think about it, you should be glad there is a rock bottom! If you didn't know God, you would be stuck in the slimy pit of mud and mire. It is hard to climb out of a pit with no bottom. Impossible even.

Rock bottom is not the worst-case scenario as a Christian. Rock bottom is when you truly find what you're made of. Praise God for giving us a solid rock!

I encourage you to make a list of all the things you can be thankful for amidst these hard times. Focus on the good. Focus on the faith.

> *I waited patiently for the Lord; He turned to me and heard my cry. He lifted me out of the slimy pit, out of the mud and mire; He set my feet on a rock and gave me a firm place to stand. He put a new song in my mouth, a hymn of praise to our God. Many will see and fear the Lord and put their trust in Him.*
>
> *—Psalms 40:1-3 NIV*

2

DO YOU WANT TO GET WELL?

Some time later, Jesus went up to Jerusalem for one of the Jewish festivals. Now there is in Jerusalem near the Sheep Gate a pool, which in Aramaic is called Bethesda and which is surrounded by five covered colonnades. Here a great number of disabled people used to lie—the blind, the lame, the paralyzed. One who was there had been an invalid for thirty-eight years. When Jesus saw him lying there and learned that he had been in this condition for a long time, he asked him, "Do you want to get well?"

"Sir," the invalid replied, "I have no one to help me into the pool when the water is stirred. While I am trying to get in, someone else goes down ahead of me."

Then Jesus said to him, "Get up! Pick up your mat and walk."

At once the man was cured; he picked up his mat and walked.

The day on which this took place was a Sabbath, and so the Jewish leaders said to the man who had been healed, "It is the Sabbath; the law forbids you to carry your mat."

But he replied, "The man who made me well said to me, 'Pick up your mat and walk.'"

So, they asked him, "Who is this fellow who told you to pick it up and walk?"

The man who was healed had no idea who it was, for Jesus had slipped away into the crowd that was there.

Later Jesus found him at the temple and said to him, "See, you are well again. Stop sinning or something worse may happen to you."

The man went away and told the Jewish leaders that it was Jesus who had made him well.

—John 5:1-15 NIV

Our dreams are there for a reason. Maybe it is a dream that we've had for a long time or maybe it is a new found dream. For many of us, having a healthy, fit body is probably a dream. It may also feel like the kind of dream that equates with winning the lottery…it's out there but we know the chances are so slim we would never get our hopes up. How sad is that? I do not believe it is many people's, if any, God-given dream to win the lottery. I do, however, believe that it is many people's God-given dream to have a healthy, fit body.

Think about it for a minute. How would it benefit God to have us be in our best physical condition? We live longer and therefore have a wider reach of witnessing. We can accomplish more good in our day because we have the energy to do so. We have an easier time encouraging people to feel and embrace the joy of the Lord because we can gain some endorphins through exercising, which lead to a better mood. You might feel that I'm reaching with these but I'm sure if you really thought about it, you could come up with some similar ones that directly apply to your life. Maybe you would feel better about going on that mission trip, speaking in public, or babysitting for a family with small children. Try journaling about this and see what comes to your mind as you write out your thoughts.

So why is it that we also feel suppressed by our dreams? You may not realize you are until you put some thought into it. What would happen if we were to ACTUALLY accomplish our dreams? Maybe we would have to give up some of our favourite excuses? "I'm just not feeling up to it today" would no longer apply because chances are when you have a healthier body, your energy will increase and your capabilities will as well. People will no longer accept the excuse you once gave. "I can't help out because my body just won't let me" will also not be usable. "I just can't do that on my own." Think about it. Your ability to be a victim will no longer exist. You will actually have to pick up your never-ending list and actually get stuff done.

At first glance, the passage I have at the top does not seem to apply to this topic, but I will never forget when I discovered the deeper meaning of Jesus asking the man if he wanted to be healed. The answer seems obvious but it is not. Jesus is asking the man if he is willing to get a job. He's asking him if he is willing to take care of himself, feed himself, contribute to society. He's asking him if he is willing to let go of his excuses and, to his fullest capability, follow Jesus by accomplishing what he was made to do. I am not downplaying his disability at all. I'm just wondering if he was truly inspired to get in the water until Jesus came into his life. No matter what our capabilities are, if they are inspired by God, they should change our motivation levels. Having a healthy body is only part of the dream. It is a stepping-stone to the bigger picture. God made us with a purpose in mind. The purpose was not to have a hot body to show off. The purpose behind having a healthy body is to do His good works that He prepared in advance for us to do (Ephesians 2:10).

There are so many mental games that we play when we try to lose weight, but what do they really matter until we decide that it is time to lose the excuses? Make a list of the excuses you could lose and how you can positively use what you have for God's plan. It's all about mindset. Change your excuses into opportunities.

3

CREATED FOR FREEDOM

You, my brothers and sisters, were called to be free. But do not use your freedom to indulge the flesh; rather, serve one another humbly in love. For the entire law is fulfilled in keeping this one command; "Love your neighbor as yourself."

—Galatians 5:13-14 NIV

The first concept I really clung to as a Christian was freedom. As someone who has always felt independent and resistant to being controlled by others, freedom was the concept I was always drawn to. To obtain the freedom to live my life in accordance to my will and values seemed like a worthy cause to strive towards. I can honestly say, however, that I never truly understood the physical, mental, and soulful freedom of Christ until I felt the humility of grace. When we fully realize the gift that grace is, we automatically gain a new appreciation for our neighbour. When we go through something that highlights our imperfect humanity, we begin to see the humanity in others as well.

We can no longer see others as a disappointment because we now know that God loves them as much as He loves us. No one is better or worse. We can no longer judge others for their actions towards us that seem less than noble because we have seen those same reactions in ourselves. Grace amplifies our compassion and empathy for others because we have truly had to receive that grace for ourselves. When we experience true grace for ourselves, we cannot help but extend it to others. Sure, we will slip and fall. We will judge and condemn. The true test of understanding grace, however, is the speed at which we can extend it to others.

Loving your neighbour as yourself will not come easily until we understand grace. We tend to lower our own self-worth by increasing our Christ-worth. And when we increase our Christ-worth, we can see our neighbour as Christ sees them. We can now love ourselves because we know our freedom in Christ was bought and paid for... just as it was for our neighbour.

What does this have to do with your weight loss journey? Everything. God extends us grace every time we slip up in our weight loss journey. We extend grace to others when they slip up in their weight loss attempts. The hard part is extending grace to ourselves when we slip up. Love yourself as you love your neighbour. Extend yourself some grace when you slip. Accept the humanity of your situation. We are not perfect but by the grace of God we can start to experience the freedom of increasing our Christ-worth.

Find some verses you can memorize and repeat in your times of judgement, both of ourselves and others. Try Matthew 22:37-38. Keep your eyes on Christ and the rest will work itself out to the glory of God in His perfect timing.

4

KEEP YOUR MIND ON THINGS FROM ABOVE

Finally, brothers and sisters, whatever is true, whatever is noble, whatever is right, whatever is pure, whatever is lovely, whatever is admirable— if anything is excellent or praiseworthy—think about such things.

—Philippians 4:8 NIV

When Jesus is telling us what the greatest commandments are, He tells us to love God with all that we are, and to love others (Mark 12:30-31). In many ways I find that so much easier to do than what the Philippians verse is telling us to do. I mean, God has given us every blessing in the heavenlies. He has died for us to give us a life of freedom. He is more than worthy of our praise. Even a good number of the people around us can be pretty easy to love…not all the time but for the most part. I sure find those two things much more manageable than trying to keep my mind on noble and pure things.

I am going to make a grand assumption that if you are reading this book, you are not trying to lose weight for the first time. I'm going to go even further to assume this isn't the second or third time. For so many people, losing weight is a lifelong journey, and I would consider them chronic dieters. Even if you have not stopped thinking about your weight for any period of time, you are probably in that category. Think about it. When was the first time you thought about losing weight? If it is more than two to three years ago, you would be a chronic dieter. The sad thing is that I have had clients who are in their 70s and have been on this journey for fifty years or so. I am going to make one more big assumption and say that the reason you could never follow through is because your brain gave up. You lost motivation. You couldn't bring your mind to make one more resolution. You could not focus on the positive aspects of your weight loss journey more than the restrictions you placed on yourself.

I get it. I never used to get it, but I certainly do now. Anyone who has not had to struggle with their weight will never understand. I never had to until recently, and let me tell you, I understand now. Let me acknowledge that it is not just laziness or junk food that led you to where you are. My guess is that the ultimate culprit is stress. We go through a trauma, we have no control in our marriage, we went through a negative sexual encounter, we lost a job, we had a close friend or family member die—the list is as long as my arm. Just know that I understand you are not just being lazy and eating too much.

Keeping our mind focused on what God has called us to is difficult. Satan knows that and abuses our weaknesses as much as he possibly can. He knows that if we don't exercise in the morning that we never will, so he puts obstacles in our way. He could even make them appear more important. He knows every trigger we have towards unhealthiness and tries to find ways to use them against us. The first thing that comes to mind when I wake up most mornings is that I need to renew my mind in Christ Jesus. Mentally, however, I actually find myself saying, *I don't want to.* It seems too hard to say the words in my head (not even out loud): *I give my weight loss journey to You, God. Please renew my mind and consistently bring my thoughts to You rather than on life and the soul-killing things of this world.* Even if I'm being super lazy or attacked, I can't get out, *Lord, help me. Lead me minute by minute today.* There is just some blockage. Mentally, I just feel exhausted even though I just opened my eyes.

My recommendation is to fight back. And yes, it will most definitely be a fight. Pray against Satan and his plans for your demise. When you aren't feeling strong enough, just start by saying the name of Jesus out loud. "Jesus, help. Jesus, fight for me." Remember that Satan cannot hear your thoughts, so speaking the name of Jesus out loud will terrify him. Throw him off guard. He knows the power that comes from that name. When you have no words of your own, quote the Bible. Memorize words of wisdom, joy, passion, purity, etc. from the Bible. I find it easier to read words that I need to be saying rather than coming up with my own on bad days. Just read them over and over again.

Be assured. We do not have this. We will not accomplish this on our own, and we never will. We've already tried that more than once.

Jesus has this. Speak the name of Jesus in all of its power, and feel the peace rush over you in that time of temptation.

Jesus.

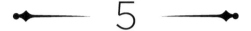

5

NOT FORSAKEN

The Lord himself goes before you and will be with you; He will never leave you nor forsake you. Do not be afraid; do not be discouraged.

—*Deuteronomy 31:8 NIV*

When it comes down to it, Christianity is so simple. It may be hard to work out in your life, but the concept behind it is so simple. Do not be afraid. Do not be discouraged. The Lord is with you. Like one day you're just going to realize, *Oh wait! Why am I afraid? God told me not to be. Okay, I'm not anymore.*

It is all about mindset. It's another reminder about how important it is to renew our minds daily…hourly even. When you feel the stress rise up, catch yourself and say,

"No! God is on my side. He will always be with me. He will be there through absolutely everything."

This is a short one today because I want you to spend the extra time memorizing this verse. Quoting scripture in your head and out loud is very important when it comes to keeping our minds focused and keeping the devil at bay. The more you say it, the more you will believe it. He will never leave you. Only someone who loves you unconditionally can say that and have it mean something powerful. People will disappoint, leave, fail, and die, but God never will. When we are struggling with our weight loss circumstances, whether we have fallen off the wagon or are trying to talk ourselves into climbing back on, God will be with us. That is something to be thankful for, and something worth turning our mindset around on.

The Lord himself goes before you and will be with you; He will never leave you nor forsake you. Do not be afraid; do not be discouraged.

—Deuteronomy 31:8 NIV

6

NOT MEANT TO
BE ALONE

*Love the Lord your God with all your heart
and with all your soul and with all your mind
and with all your strength. The second is this;
"Love your neighbor as yourself" There is no
commandment greater than these.*

—Mark 12:30-31 NIV

When you think about being alone and what God has planned for you, you may not think of this verse. The reason I wanted to highlight this verse in this context is that aside from loving God with everything that you are, you are meant to love people…which means you are not meant to be alone.

Even though you are unique, I want you to know that you are not alone. One of the biggest lies the enemy puts out there is that you are the only one going through this, and you should deal with it alone. I think we can all agree that we are not alone in our struggle to lose weight. Believing that we are keeps us small and powerless. Your journey will not be like anyone else's, but that does not mean we cannot lend or accept support as we move forward. We are meant to live in community, thrive in community, and depend on community in the highs and lows of our lives.

Does this mean we cannot pursue goals on our own? Absolutely not. I would recommend telling at least one other person about your intentions to lose weight. You do not have to do this, but it may help you with accountability or even just prayer support. Knowing that there is someone out there on your side is encouraging. If you do not feel like there is anyone in your life who can lend that kind of non-judgmental support, pray that God will bring someone into your life who truly understands what you are going through. They might be praying to find someone like you right now too! Make a list of potential people who you could tell, or decide to pray every day for God to bring someone to you.

You can only truly understand someone else when you go through something similar yourself. This is why, as a Christian, one of our greatest assets is going through hard times. Offering the gift of understanding to someone else is priceless, and it is strong enough to help you both find a new way to move through a seemingly impossible situation.

Love God first. Love others next. Let them love you.

7

PRESS ON TOWARDS THE GOAL

Further, my brothers and sisters, rejoice in the Lord! It is no trouble for me to write the same things to you again, and it is a safeguard for you. Watch out for those dogs, those evildoers, those mutilators of the flesh. For it is we who are the circumcision, we who serve God by his Spirit, who boast in Christ Jesus, and who put no confidence in the flesh—though I myself have reasons for such confidence.

If someone else thinks they have reasons to put confidence in the flesh, I have more: circumcised on the eighth day, of the people of Israel, of the tribe of Benjamin, a Hebrew of Hebrews; in regard to the law, a Pharisee; as for zeal, persecuting the church; as for righteousness based on the law, faultless.

But whatever were gains to me, I now consider loss for the sake of Christ. What is more, I consider everything a loss because of the surpassing worth of knowing Christ Jesus my Lord, for whose sake I have lost all things. I consider them garbage, that I may gain Christ and be found in Him, not having a righteousness of my own that comes from the law, but that which is through faith in Christ—the righteousness that comes from God on the basis of faith. I want to know Christ—yes, to know the power of His resurrection and participation in His sufferings, becoming like Him in his death, and so, somehow, attaining to the resurrection from the dead.

Not that I have already obtained all this, or have already arrived at my goal, but I press on to take hold of that for which Christ Jesus took hold of me. Brothers and sisters, I do not consider myself yet to have taken hold of it. But one thing I do: Forgetting what is behind and straining toward what is ahead, I press on toward the goal to win the prize for which God has called me heavenward in Christ Jesus.

—Philippians 3:1-14 NIV

A few things jump out to me as I read this. First off is that we have no reason to put our trust in the flesh—in our humanity. I'm guessing that if you are reading this devotional for the reason it was intended (to help you gain God's perspective on your health priorities), then you have put your trust in your flesh more than once. It's so easy to do. When it comes to our health goals, it's as easy as thinking that all we need to do is follow a certain diet and we'll achieve what we desire…and yet we try to do this over and over again. We try doing the exact same thing over and over again thinking that THIS time it will have a different outcome. Does anyone know what the definition of insanity is? Yup. That's it. Now, do I think that everyone out there doing this is insane? Obviously not. I do, however, think we are putting our faith in our flesh rather than our Savior sometimes. Now I know there are those of you out there who would say that you have tried to involve God in your weight loss or health journey but it still didn't work. Did you ever think that maybe during those times that He just changed what the outcome would be? It was His outcome rather than yours? Just think about that for a moment.

I have tested so many "diets" (either in real life or in my head) that I know for a fact that I have chosen not to devote my food and exercise plans to God. Sometimes I do, but sometimes I just don't think of it. I think of it as being separate or maybe just overlook it. Again, I'm not condemning anyone here—no one other than myself that is. But maybe you can relate. I'm thinking you probably can. We are busy. We are lazy. We are easily distracted. The list goes on and on. But if we think about the things in our lives that hold the top spot on our priority list, they should get the most attention from us. The most devotion. And yet, as we all know, those are the things that tend to slip our attention more than they should.

We see this over and over in the Bible. Real people experiencing the same problems we do. God chose people of weak faith, weak bodies, weak minds, and weak life experience to do the most important jobs for Him. He chose people who appear weak to those around them to show them His infinite love. Does that mean we are all a bunch of weaklings? Again, no. It means that if we take a good solid look at our flesh, we know that we would be truly nothing without God. Just dirt.

The next thing I notice about the scripture is that the sooner we realize our flesh is fallible, the sooner we get to grasp the goodness God has called us to—communion with Him. Not all the actions we can do for and in Him, but Him. He is the prize. He is everything. So often we focus on everything but Him while trying to serve Him. We focus on our own healing. We focus on how God can bring about amazing change. We focus on the people we can serve. We focus on the spiritual realms that both help and hinder us. We focus on the mission God has called us to. All of these things are not bad. God would never say that. He created all of them for a purpose. But when we seek to serve, heal, change, and understand, we forget WHO God is. We burn out because our fountain isn't overflowing with the God we love and chose to follow. We need to commit to God himself and trust that the rest will fall into His hands.

Lastly, what I notice is the goal: *I press on towards the goal for which God has called me heavenward*. I forget the failures of my past and look to my future. I look to the God that has given me a purpose-driven life. A purpose to strive for Him. When that becomes our purpose, the rest just overflows. The serving. The changing. The healing. If our number one goal is God, the rest will fall into place.

Before I end this, I want you to know that because you haven't previously succeeded in your health and wellness goals does NOT mean you do not love your God. Not even a little bit. The fact that you are still trying means you have hope. And where does our hope come from? God. The beginning and the end. The one that helps us pick ourselves up and keep trying. The one who loved you SO MUCH that He sent His only son to die on a cross for you. And, thank goodness, there is NOTHING you can do to stop Him from loving you that much. He is so proud of you and all that you try to accomplish. It is when you lose hope that you know you have fallen away. It is when you lose faith that you quit getting back up. It is when you start to feel emotionless that you lose love. But just remember "these three remain: faith, hope, and love. But the greatest of these is love" (1 Cor 13:13). "Love the Lord your God with all your heart and with all your soul and with all your strength" (Duet 6:5). When all we can do is love God, it will always be enough. If we have to stay in bed all day, but still love? That is enough. Our God is the best Father we could ever hope for and will never, ever stop loving us. If the best you can do on any one day is submit to accepting His love, that is enough. You are enough. Press on to knowing Him better. He is worth it.

Start making a list that is to be ongoing throughout this devotional about all that you can learn about who God is. This can be something to look back on when you need to be reminded who you are putting your trust in.

8

TIRED OF TRYING

*Come to me, all you who are weary and burdened,
and I will give you rest. Take my yoke upon you
and learn from me, for I am gentle and humble
in heart, and you will find rest for your souls. For
my yoke is easy and my burden is light.*

—Matthew 11:28-30 NIV

Is it just me, or are there more days like this than energetic ones? I am convinced that the number one way the devil interferes in our life, goals, and desires is by killing our drive. He makes everything seem hopeless. He questions our intentions, asking if it is even worth it to try so hard to accomplish something. These are the times when we fall off the wagon and it can take days, weeks, months or even years to get back on and try again. Achieving what we want—what we know God wants for us—can be exhausting. It's not a continuously forward motion. HOPEFULLY, it's two steps forward, one step back, but it may feel like we are moving backwards more than forwards sometimes.

The main question to ask yourself is: Is this a time to rest and recoup or is it a time to fight? Sometimes our version of fighting will be a quiet one. It will be more reading the Bible and more purposeful prayer. Maybe it will be reading a story that inspires you. We need to follow Jesus' instructions and go to Him. How can we turn being weary and burdened into something positive? We take the yoke of Jesus and learn from Him. He will, in turn, generously give us rest for our souls. Use this time to focus on the Giver of Life. Go for a walk. Breathe deeply and be thankful for the blessings in your life. Pray that tomorrow or at a time not too long from now, your energy will be restored and your passion reignited for the desires He placed in your heart.

Take the time to write out this scripture and memorize it so it can be recited when these times come upon you.

The Lord is my shepherd; I shall not want.

He makes me lie down in green pastures; He leads me beside quiet waters.

He restores my soul; He guides me in the paths of righteousness for His name's sake.

Even though I walk through the valley of the shadow of death, I fear no evil, for You are with me; Your rod and Your staff, they comfort me.

You prepare a table before me in the presence of my enemies; You have anointed my head with oil; my cup overflows.

Surely goodness and loving kindness will follow me all the days of my life, and I will dwell in the house of the Lord forever.

—Psalms 23 NAS

9

WHAT ARE YOUR GREATEST STRENGTHS?

Sometimes we are so focused on the negative parts of ourselves that we forget there are so many things we are good at. I have had so many clients come to me that are so very successful in their lives…except in weight loss. It seems to be the one thing they just can't figure out, and it tends to overtake their mindset so they cannot even appreciate the successes they have had in the rest of their lives. It is such a sad situation and one that our enemy uses against us all the time.

> *Be alert and of sober mind. Your enemy the devil prowls around like a roaring lion looking for someone to devour.*
>
> *—1 Peter 5:8 NIV*

There are so many different ways our strengths can be used against us by the enemy. He could use them to invoke pride, pressure, or tunnel vision. He could promote idolatry or cause you to have an insatiable hunger for more and more success. Our strengths could also be used to overlook our weaknesses. Being overweight is a major weakness for many, and when we are strong in other things, we may just leave that one weakness alone. Being overweight is not just a weakness that sits and stays. It is usually one that wears us down over time. It is one that causes many diseases, symptoms, and health issues. It is something that can put you out of commission well before your time.

Does that mean it is bad to have strengths? Obviously not. God created us in His own image and, therefore, gave us many strengths that are unique to us. It would be ungodly to ignore our strengths just in case they could be used against us. What is more important is to use our strengths to help us overcome our weaknesses. If you are reading this, I will assume that your struggle with weight is one of your weaknesses. Use your strength of reading to memorize verses so you can quote them at the devil as he tries to make you forget what is really important. Use your gift of prayer to put up a hedge of protection around yourself and your health. Use your authority in Christ to command angels to bring your prayer requests to the minds of people who know your struggles. Use your connection with friends and family to gain support for your mission. Most of all, use the love Christ gave us to help us understand deep in our hearts that He wants the very best for us. He wants us to love Him and love others.

Just know that if you are a Christian, the enemy WILL try to put you out of commission. Being attacked by the devil is one big pat on the back. It means that you are on the right track and you need to fight even harder to accomplish what you are trying to do. It means that if you can accomplish this task, others will be saved or pushed in that direction. Others will join our side. Others will see the truth and come to believe. Try to see the bigger picture. Try to put aside vanity and look to the cross. Know that in that cross, the war has been won. It cannot be un-won. With that as your cornerstone, you can accomplish anything. Don't give up! Keep putting your complete strength in God knowing that you can crush your enemy with a spoken word.

10

A PEACE THAT TRANSCENDS

Do not be anxious about anything, but in every situation, by prayer and petition, with thanksgiving, present your requests to God. And the peace of God, which transcends all understanding, will guard your hearts and your minds in Christ Jesus.

—Philippians 4:6-7 NIV

*D*on't *be anxious about anything* is such a simple command that can be very hard to follow. Just don't worry about it. We all know that worrying doesn't change anything except for our demeanour...how we treat people, how we react to situations, and how we choose to proceed with the problem at hand. What I mean is that worrying does not change the fact that we still have to deal with a problem. It just changes how we deal with that problem.

Worrying is not from God and, therefore, the symptoms of worry are not at all beneficial to us. Worry causes a lack of peace in the form of restlessness, lack of sleep, anxiety, depression, lack of patience, and the list goes on. According to Paul in Ephesians 6 when he speaks about the armour of God, we are to always have our feet ready with the gospel of peace. That means that no matter what problems we face, we can go into it knowing that God is always in control and ready to help us navigate the problems we are attempting to resolve. The peace that Paul speaks about here is beyond our understanding. How can we feel peaceful when our world is falling down around us? Because we trust that God will be with us. If we fully trust God we can be thankful in any situation. When we are thankful, it triggers peace because it comes full circle in reminding us that we know we can trust God.

Depending on your situation, I hope you can somehow muster some trust or thankfulness. If we are really focused on God, we will never have a hard time that cannot be countered with thankfulness. In the very least, which is actually the very most, we can be thankful that Christ saved us from our sins. If you can trust nothing else, trust that. Meditate on that. Focus your energies on that. Such a great sacrifice made it easy to always have something to be thankful for, and instead of going into a downward worry spiral, you can rise with the winds of thanksgiving to the higher ground of peace.

The journey to a healthier body will probably not be easy. It will be a fight every day to renew our minds and trust that God is in control of this. But when you trust God is in control of your body, you can be thankful for a God who cares about your cares and be peaceful with wherever this journey takes you. Remember that God does not have any use for a beach body. He does have use for a healthy, long-living, Christ-filled body and soul to bring the good news of peace and thanksgiving to everyone around you. Your mission, should you choose to accept it, is peace.

11

A GRANDMOTHER'S WISDOM

Recently, one of my most favourite people in the world passed away. My grandma. She was someone who was always there when I called. She knew my voice before there was video calling or call display. Even in her last days when her thoughts weren't always so clear, she STILL knew it was me calling her after I said, "Hello." What a blessing to have people like that in our lives.

My grandma was a woman of God who longed to go home for quite some time before she got there. She had dreams of my grandpa meeting her at the gates saying, *What took you so long?* She was a woman who read her Bible and made notes in it everywhere. She put notes paperclipped in, as well as in every spare space you could find. Her Bible was worn out in the best possible way. While going through some of her writings I found the piece below. I can take no credit for what you are about

36

to read, but I am confident she would be excited to know her words were being passed on.

> *And we know that all things work together for good to them that love God, to them who are called according to his purpose.*
>
> —*Romans 8:28 KJV*

As per Grandma:

This is one of God's promises we can rest on when the world around us has fallen apart, a promise we can believe and trust when we do not understand. Days of adversity as well as days of prosperity can bring us blessings if we let them.

God says He will let all things work together for our good. When we let God enter the picture, He will take all our experiences and work them out for our good. The Bible says "all things," not "some things" or "most things," but all. Every one.

We wonder how the great tragedy or heartache or pain we're experiencing can bring good to us. And the isolated experiences themselves may not be good, or bring good to us. But God will work them together for our good.

God will do all of this for *those who love God* and *those who are called according to His purpose.* We may not know how good comes from our adversities, but to know that good does come should be sufficient. Not all things are good, but He will transform them for our good. God is behind His promise to make it good.

I encourage you to find a version of this verse that really reads well for you. They are all similar, but find the translation that you want to memorize and repeat in those hard times.

12

DEEPER ISSUES

So do not fear, for I am with you; do not be dismayed, for I am your God. I will strengthen you and help you; I will uphold you with my righteous right hand.

—Isaiah 41:10 NIV

Everyone has a reason for gaining weight, and it can be a very powerful tool in your weight loss journey to identify it. I have a few theories to help give you an idea of where to start looking.

The first theory is that you gained weight for a very specific reason, even though you may not have known it at the time. Many people gain weight as a form of protection. Anyone who has been assaulted either physically, sexually, mentally, or emotionally has possibly used their weight as a means to either protect themselves or gain some sort of control over their situation.

My second theory is that you have had some form of health problem that has either affected your ability to keep a homeostatic weight or has made you take medications that cause weight gain.

My third theory is that you have gone through some extremely stressful or traumatic situations either continuously or that have had lasting effects on you. I would consider a stressful job, living conditions, or relationships, deaths, break-ups, etc. in this category.

The fourth theory is that it is a combination of the first three plus a few other side orders of personal failures and letdowns, as well as just getting older.

It can be a very powerful thing to identify the reason you have gained weight. I encourage you to spend some time thinking about it. It's a bit tricky to follow it back to the exact source, but I want you to think about when you started feeling like you had a problem with your weight. Usually you will associate it with some life event. When you can pinpoint that, look back further. Did you have that issue before then? Do some soul searching. Take your time. Journal it out.

Putting a "face" to your problem will help you be able to move forward. For many, it is actually scary to move forward because it means opening yourself up again to whatever made you gain the weight to begin with. It can open up other problems that may not have been there before. It can force you to deal with some very hard emotions.

You are not alone. Listen to the All-Powerful God of the Angel Armies when He says in Isaiah 41:10, "So do not fear, for I am with you; do not be dismayed, for I am your God. I will strengthen you and help you; I will uphold you with my righteous right hand."

You either trust all or none of the Bible. If you believe it is true, then you can trust that God will always be with you, He will always strengthen you, and He will always uphold you. Trust in that as you work through some of your deeper issues.

13

I THINK,
THEREFORE I AM

All of our fears are sinful, and we create our own fears by refusing to nourish ourselves in our faith. How can anyone who identifies with Jesus Christ suffer from doubt or fear? Our lives should be an absolute hymn of praise resulting from perfect, irrepressible, triumphant belief.

—Oswald Chambers

I love Oswald Chambers. He appeals to the blunt, honest side of me. When I first read this quote, I was so inspired with how black and white it seemed. If you love and follow Christ, you should not have fear or doubt in your life. End of story. The more I read it, however, the more I questioned putting it in this devotional. When you are going through a weight loss struggle (or any struggle) there are times you doubt you can do it. It just seems so harsh. How can we praise all the time? And then I found this verse:

> *Why, my soul, are you downcast? Why so disturbed within me? Put your hope in God, for I will yet praise him, my Savior and my God.*
>
> —*Psalms 42:11 NIV*

I love King David's self-talk. I love that he is questioning his own attitude. He talks to his soul as if it is a separate entity. Why are you so blue? Put your hope in God, silly soul! He will never let you down! So often we lose perspective of the big picture. We put our focus on how our dietary restrictions make us feel deprived. We focus on how we have failed multiple weight loss attempts before. Have you ever heard the saying, "I think, therefore I am"? Well, like many other common sayings, it comes from a Bible verse:

> *For as he thinks in his heart, so is he.*
>
> —*Proverbs 23:7 NKJV*

If we believe we will fail, we will. If we believe we feel deprived, we will be. But if we change our thoughts, it brings such freedom and joy. I know I cannot lose weight on my own, BUT I know God can do anything, therefore, I release my weight loss journey into His perfect hands.

Praise God that I can release all my cares onto Him! All I have to do is commit my ways to God and my life will be full of joy, praise, and a grateful heart. Will it be easy? Nothing worth doing ever is. But if you are persistent and motivated, God will direct your journey.

I encourage you to write out your own self-talk. Here is mine right now and it just happens to have a little rhyme in it for fun:

I will do my devotions.
I will exercise.
I will eat healthy.
I will drink water.
I will write.
My body will change.
My books will sell.
My God will be there through it all.

I also really like this one:
Water is life.
Exercise is strength.
Mindset moves mountains.

Yours does not have to be poetic. Just honest.

14

SIMPLE CONCEPT, DIFFICULT TO EXECUTE

Trust in the Lord with all your heart and lean not on your own understanding; in all your ways submit to Him, and he will make your paths straight.

—Proverbs 3:5-6 NIV

I've heard these verses since my younger years in Sunday School, and even though it is a simple concept, it gets harder to truly grasp as I get older. It is true that, in some ways, children have us beat in terms of "getting God". Why do we lose that simple faith? It comes to us inherently. We are born trusting our parents. It is us as the grown-ups that make them lose their simple faith. We let them down with our own humanity. The only thing we can continue to try and impart into them is that even though we are not perfect, God is, and they will always be able to trust Him.

But what about now? We are older, wiser, and more worldly. We have good reason not to trust those around us. Even those of us who try to keep the faith in humankind are constantly disappointed. Not only that, we continually let ourselves down. We make poor decisions. We fail at all aspects of life. We have no will-power. It's funny how we can let ourselves down over and over again and yet we continue to put our trust in ourselves rather than in God.

Remember the definition of insanity? Doing the same thing over and over again expecting a different outcome. Let's stop the insanity!

Even though the most logical solution may seem like trusting ourselves to make wise choices, when we don't involve God in them, we are setting ourselves up for failure. Now I know the argument you're going to propose: God gave me common sense and a gut, why can't I follow that? You definitely can, as long as you have committed your common sense and gut to God. See where I'm going with this? God gave us so many gifts to use for His glory, but if we do not commit those gifts back to Him, we are like an empty vase. We have the structure to be useful, but are we actually being useful if we're not being used? Does that make sense? We have everything we need in Christ, but if we choose not to give it back to Him, is it really worth using?

What do you need to commit to God? Figure that out for yourself today and put a plan in place to help keep you in check. Mindset is the hardest for me. It can kill my goals faster than anything else. I try to commit my mind to God and repeat the proverb above when I feel resistance. I encourage you to do the same.

I don't know about you but I'd much rather have a straight path than a curvy one. It's so much less dramatic and time consuming. When we put all of our efforts into just loving God and putting our full heart into trusting Him, the rest will fall into place. The goals we have, if God given, will be achieved. The desires in our hearts are satisfied when we place them in God's hands. Thankfully, those same hands are attached to His ever-loving arms for holding all of us if we would submit to Him completely. Trust in the Lord, people; it is the best thing we could ever do for our health and well-being. The very worst that could happen is that our goals are set aside for more important things, and we won't care because God will have replaced them with His own goals. Focus on the bigger picture. Focus on God. Our goals mean nothing if we cannot put our all into loving the Creator of all.

15

SOARING IS PREFERABLE TO SLITHERING

But they that wait upon the Lord shall renew their strength; they shall mount up with wings as eagles; they shall run, and not be weary; and they shall walk, and not faint.

—Isaiah 40:31 KJV

The Lord God said to the serpent, "Because you have done this, cursed are you above all livestock and above all beasts of the field; on your belly you shall go, and dust you shall eat all the days of your life."

—Genesis 3:14 ESV

I've never thought to compare an eagle to a snake until this moment, but it is such a useful description to picture of how different our lives could be because of one decision.

Throughout time, and across cultures, people have seen eagles as a symbol of beauty, pride, determination, bravery, courage, honour, and grace. It flies higher than any other bird and has the sharpest vision out there. It is used as an example of what we should strive to be—someone who is admired and an example of truth and honesty.

A snake, however, according to the Bible, is a cursed animal. Cursed above all the other animals on the earth. It must look up from the dust to everything and everyone. It seems conniving and dishonest and manipulative. It needs to fight for everything it gets and will always be at the foot of the more powerful man.

Thanks to Jesus Christ, we do not need to live a cursed life but rather one of blessings on high. Because of His sacrifice and ascension, we have the Holy Spirit within us and are able to commune with God, anytime and anywhere. We have the ability to hope in the Lord. When we get down on ourselves, the world around us, or humankind, we can bring those concerns to God. When we feel discouraged and weary about our goals, we can bring those concerns to God. Not only will He lift us up mentally but also physically. He will give us the means to keep going. This means to *run and not grow weary, walk and not faint.* We have the means to accomplish our God-given goals, but we need to remember that it is going to be achieved via God's means. It means we have a choice. Choose to fly. Choose to be thankful for the many blessings we have been given. Choose to choose. Only you have the power to choose how you react. Don't let yourself be drawn into slithering by laziness. Choose to fly.

Some people overlook the beauty and imagination of children's TV shows, but, thankfully, I have two toddlers who love a popular Christian vegetable cartoon. At the end of an episode where it shows kids just how important we are to God, just how we are created to use our gifts for Him and not to worry about what other people think about them, it ends with this saying, "He wants you to sing, He wants you to paint, and He wants you to soar." It makes me tear up every time. God, our Father, wants us to soar.

16

PRAISE BE TO GOD

Praise be to the God and Father of our Lord Jesus Christ, the Father of compassion and the God of all comfort, who comforts us in all our troubles, so that we can comfort those in any trouble with the comfort we ourselves receive from God. For just as we share abundantly in the sufferings of Christ, so also our comfort abounds through Christ. If we are distressed, it is for your comfort and salvation; if we are comforted, it is for your comfort, which produces in you patient endurance of the same sufferings we suffer. And our hope for you is firm, because we know that just as you share in our sufferings, so also you share in our comfort.

—2 Corinthians 1:3-7 NIV

I think this verse says it all. God gives us comfort so we can also offer it to others. He allows our sufferings so we can comfort those going through the same thing. For those in our lives who do not know Christ like we do, we could be their only way of accepting God's comfort. Sharing comfort with fellow Christians is also important. Let us not make the mistake of thinking that sharing comfort is whining and complaining about our situation. It means you get to vent, you get to pray together, and it means you get to come up with a plan. It means you can rest in the comfort of God together. Remember that the negative thoughts we dwell on will not lead us to higher ground. Dwelling on the comfort of God's love is uplifting.

If you don't know this song, I encourage you to look it up and listen to it. Get it stuck in your head. Use it as your form of meditation today.

What a Friend We Have in Jesus

What a friend we have in Jesus,
All our sins and griefs to bear!
And what a privilege to carry
Everything to God in prayer!

Oh, what peace we often forfeit,
Oh, what needless pain we bear,
All because we do not carry
Everything to God in prayer!

Have we trials and temptations?
Is there trouble anywhere?
We should never be discouraged,
Take it to the Lord in prayer.

Can we find a friend so faithful
Who will all our sorrows share?
Jesus knows our every weakness,
Take it to the Lord in prayer.

Are we weak and heavy-laden,
Cumbered with a load of care?
Precious Savior, still our refuge,
Take it to the Lord in prayer;

Do thy friends despise, forsake thee?
Take it to the Lord in prayer;
In His arms He'll take and *shield thee,*
Thou wilt find a solace there.

Songwriters: Charles Crozat Converse, Joseph Scriven

17

ARMOUR OF GOD

Finally, be strong in the Lord and in the strength of his might. Put on the whole armour of God, that you may be able to stand against the schemes of the devil. For we do not wrestle against the flesh and blood, but against the rulers, against the authorities, against the cosmic powers over this present darkness, against the spiritual forces of evil in the heavenly places. Therefore, take up the whole armour of God, that you may be able to withstand in the evil day, and having done all, to stand firm. Stand therefore, having fastened on the belt of truth, and having put on the breastplate of righteousness, and, as shoes for your feet having put on the readiness given by the gospel of peace. In all circumstances take up the shield of faith, with which you can extinguish all the flaming darts of the evil one; and take the helmet of salvation, and the sword of the spirit,

*which is the word of God, praying at all times in
the spirit, with all prayer and supplication.*

—*Ephesians 6:10-18 ESV*

I've always been a big "fan" of the armour of God. I just like picturing a scene in *The Lord of the Rings* when Théoden, King of Rohan, is in a room making a bit of a defeated speech before the battle of Helm's Deep commences. He was wondering how the world came to the point where he had to force boys and men to fight a huge army of, basically, hate. How can you fight such hatred? He keeps speaking while one of his men dresses him in his armour. Fortunately, later in the battle, when it looks like all is lost, he chooses to take up his sword and ride out in battle. If it is to be his end, he wants to go down fighting for what is right and what is good: Love. Only love can truly combat hatred.

But you know what the catch is?

You have to be prepared. You can't just wait for the battle to come to you and THEN get prepared. You have to be ready for it at any time. You can't ride out with your sword if you forgot it in the castle vault.

Up until recently I just liked reciting these components of armour to myself in the morning. Like when I did, I knew I would be protected throughout the day from attacks. Then I had an insight. Maybe it's just me and

I'm the only one who never caught on to this, but hear me out. How can we *fasten the belt of truth* if we lie all the time? How can we *put on the breastplate of righteousness* if we are not practising living according to God's will? How can we wear the *shoes of the readiness of the gospel of peace* if we are going around causing confrontations? How can we take up the *shield of faith* if we have no faith? How can we put on *the helmet of salvation* if we are not living like a saved child of God? And how can we wield our *swords of the spirit, which is the word of God*, if we can't quote any verses from it?

I used to think I just needed to say these things every morning to cover myself, but I do not believe that anymore. It's not something we have to say. It's something we have to be. We need to become our armour. It's like exercising. We need to build our muscles and let it show we take care of ourselves. We need to surround ourselves with our armour. We need to learn to practice truth. We need to live according to God's will. We need to exude peace. We need to go through every day knowing and believing that God has our back. We need to memorize scripture so that it has a chance to come to mind when the devil comes prowling. And God needs to always be the first response. He needs to be in our mind all day. We need to talk and pray to Him throughout our day. Don't ever think that some care or concern we have is too small. He wants all of us always. I knew I had a win in this category when I started talking to God about sports during big games… Do I need to pray about that? Absolutely not. But I do (and then I tell Him it's okay if my team doesn't win because it doesn't really matter) because when He is my first instinct, that is what comes out sometimes. Try to work this into your day everyday. We have the best listener with us all the time.

What does this have to do with a healthy lifestyle? It means we need to get our focus on the right things. Who cares about our physical health if our spiritual health is lacking? When we take our eyes off of our well intended goals and focus them on the God (who put those goals in our heads), things may just start to come together. Or they won't. Frustrating as it sounds, it's a great thing. If our eyes are on God and things don't happen as we want them to, then we are okay with it because it is no longer our first concern. It is now more important to exude the qualities of Christ and learn to accept the circumstances He has given us. Sometimes our greatest weaknesses (our struggle with weight) are used as God's greatest strengths. When someone is struggling through a weight loss journey, who do you want to hear from? Someone who has it together all the time? Or someone who has experience and vulnerability, which could be the one thing that a very closed-off person needs to see in order to open up. I'm not saying this is the case for everyone. What I am saying is if we focus on God, He will use our journey the way He wants. And the more we grow in faith, the more we trust Him with this task.

18

GOOD PLANS

"For I know the plans I have for you," declares the Lord, "plans to prosper you and not to harm you, plans to give you hope and a future."

—Jeremiah 29:11 NIV

We make our plans, but the Lord determines our steps.

—Proverbs 16:9 NLT

Listen to advice and accept discipline, and at the end you will be counted among the wise. Many are the plans in a person's heart, but it is the Lord's purpose that prevails.

—Proverbs 19:20-21 NIV

The list of verses that can confirm this same thing over and over again are endless. The Lord is everything. He knows everything. He has it all planned out and will determine the steps we need to get there if we follow His directions every step of the way. His plans are good and are meant for our own good.

This is all well and fine but we tend to think big picture. We want to know the end game before we get there. We want to know what all of these little "nothing" steps lead up to. What is the grand finale? Have you ever thought that if you heard what your grand finale was before the time was right, that you'd go running for the hills? I remember hearing a story about a church family who were firmly planted in their life in Canada. They loved their jobs and were doing exactly what God had called them to. They had always stated that they were so glad their calling was "here at home." One thing led to another and while following God's plan they first stepped into more of a leadership role at church. Then they did outreach within the city. Eventually they felt called overseas to plant a church. They were not at all hesitant when the time came because God had taken them step by step through HIS plan and led them right into a situation they never thought they'd be involved in.

As I mentioned in the Introduction, I used to journal a lot, but I thought it of more as thinking as opposed to writing; a way to process my life. I've come to a greater understanding of my life because of it. When it came to doing it as a part of my career, however, I totally rejected it…until I didn't. God took me through a lifetime of ups and downs so I would be ready to share my knowledge with you. Writing became a natural progression and one that brings a smile to my face (and maybe a little smirk to God's). He always knew how my heart would conform to His will and how I would love it. Again, I just love how God and I communicate. He just meets me on my level and slowly moves me towards Himself…sometimes with a little sarcasm just for fun.

That's a long way to say that God has a plan. If He had told me about it years in advance, I would've run the other direction. God's way is perfect though, and He gave me one step at a time. He didn't let me get ahead of myself. He just kept affirming where I was. There were many bumps along the way, but I certainly do not count them as loss because experience is what has connected me to people. Have you ever tried to talk to someone about weight loss who has never had a weight concern in their life? The answers are sometimes insensitive and even somewhat rude. Have you ever had someone tell you in the depths of depression to just pull yourself together? Ignorance. Count your experiences as a blessing. They help you love and serve better.

Think of God as your car GPS. It doesn't give you every direction right away. In a trip across the country you'd never remember and you would probably get lost. But, like God, it tells you when to make a right turn and what off-ramp to take at the right time. Are you uncertain if you're on the right track? Well, what does a GPS do when you're going the right way? Nothing. It's silent. Keep following God's direction for your life and He will let you know when it's time to make a change. If He is silent just keep plugging away and trusting His perfect purpose for your life. His plans are good and made to help you prosper.

Can you sense a pattern in your life? Maybe writing it down could help you process too. I have to admit that since I've had kids my journaling has taken on a different form. I think it all out and then write down the main points. I have time to think during the day but not much time to just sit and write. Now I just write it out in bullet points. Sometimes it only makes it onto a notes app on my phone but it has the same effect. Find something that works for you. Even bullet points can show a trend.

19

THE JOY OF THE LORD IS MY STRENGTH

I like to think of myself as a highly intuitive person. I can pick up on people's personalities quickly and feel that I can get a good read of a person. If you can believe it, I totally knew what my kids' main personality traits would be before they were born. My son would be easily excitable and my daughter, determined. I was very right. When it comes to this devotional, I also like to just feel my way around to see what seems right. When it comes down to it, it's not anything to do with my intuition but more about what God puts on my mind when the time is right. When I made the very messy outline for this devotional, this topic wasn't on it at all…but it just came to me now. When I looked up the verse that went along with this saying, I had to laugh.

Nehemiah said, "Go and enjoy choice food and sweet drinks, and send some to those who have

> *nothing prepared. This day is holy to our Lord. Do*
> *not grieve, for the joy of the Lord is your strength."*

> —*Nehemiah 8:10 NIV*

What a sense of humour God has. Really? He's telling me to share Nehemiah's exhortation to *Enjoy the choice food and sweet drinks* in a devotional precisely geared towards health and wellness? Come on! Who doesn't want to obey that command?

Now I am no theologian by any means, but I do know how important it is to read scripture in context. The funny thing about this situation is that I think God means for us to not overthink this. God created so much of our world to be enjoyed. He never meant for us to go outside and loathe the fresh air or get annoyed by the breeze coming off the ocean. He meant for us to take in deep breaths even in our times of trouble and know that we can find joy in the small things.

This is how we are meant to eat as well, so let's take this as literally as we can. What do you think of when you think of choice food? I think of a lovely barbecued steak and vegetables with a baked potato on the side. Or maybe a bowl of fresh pasta with freshly roasted vegetables and chicken. What I mean to say is that when I think of "choice food", I do not think of fast food. I do not think of something from a store that is open 24/7. I do not think of something that comes in a package with ingredients that sound more like scientific dribble than something edible. Choice food takes time and care to create.

Now the "sweet drinks." Honestly the first thing that comes to my mind when I think of sweet drinks is a pop, iced tea or lemonade. I am quite certain that is not what He meant, however. When it is hot outside, there is nothing that will quench your thirst better than a drink of fresh, cold water. I am reminded of a time when my husband went quadding in the mountains and he came upon a trickle of a creek that turned into a stream and then into a waterfall. He thought it was the best water he had ever tasted so he emptied his water bottle and brought me back some. It really was good. When something is fresh and straight from the source, it is an experience. It satisfies in more ways than one.

I think God meant for us to enjoy our food and drink. But even more than that, He wants us to think of our bodies as a temple and to nourish that temple with food and drink that will sustain us, and make us into the people He wants us to be. On that note, I believe there is a time for everything food-wise. There is a time to feast and a time to fast. But for the most part, we need to think of and eat in a way that will satisfy our needs.

People often ask me which diet plans I support. I tell them I support whatever works for them and help them pursue it in the healthiest way possible. How is it possible to think that one diet is right for everyone? That's just ridiculous. We are as different as the diets we should be consuming. If I gave you the healthiest diet in the world but you couldn't follow it, what is the point? On a similar note, I always say that if I were to write my own diet book it would be the shortest one ever. Lucky for you, I will let you in on my secret:

> "Eat real food. Cut processed foods." That's it. There's my book.

This "secret" is inclusive of any type of dietary needs without limiting you to any certain thing. It's genius… in my opinion. We make food into an enemy, when it is actually the very thing that keeps us alive.

Just a quick note on the middle part of that verse where we are told to share with those who have nothing. As much as it is great to take that literally and share our food with others, I think a big part of it is also just to get outside of ourselves. When we go on a diet, that's all we think about. What if we focused on a bigger picture? The other part about not grieving is something we really tend to focus on when we go on a diet. We grieve the things we "can't have." The thing is, if we were to choose a diet full of variety and fresh, healthy food, the only feeling we should have is thankfulness. Again, let's get outside of our flesh and focus on what is really important.

The other thing we need to focus on is *the joy of the Lord.* Let's think like a parent for a second since God is the ultimate Father. As a parent of toddlers, one of the hardest things to see is your child hurting. But the joy? Oh, the joy that comes when they fall in love with life and experiences and friends and family and the world around them. Our Lord created us to be His joy. He created us to love us. The ironic thing is that if we work that in reverse, we are the ones full of joy. When we take pleasure in our Saviour, we have true joy. Happiness comes and goes. Joy lasts a lifetime. When we take joy in the One who created joy, we will never go wrong.

Now let's take that one step further and add in the strength. *The joy of the Lord is our strength.* Our flesh is nothing but weak. It is feeble. It has no will-power. Thank God, that as Christians, we have more to rely on than just ourselves. Let's rewrite that phrase:

The joy of the Lord is us, His children, taking joy in Him. It is us realizing that if we are to do anything truly purposeful in this life, we must put our complete focus on the One who gave us purpose in the first place. Our strength is knowing that our Father is on our side. Our strength comes from loving our Saviour and being insatiable when it comes to knowing Him.

When our focus is on our Saviour, we will never go wrong. It is whether we can pick up on the outcomes that He is showing us rather than the one we have planned for ourselves. Let's start by being thankful, which should lead us to being joyful in the strength and power of our Lord.

20

CRUSHED IN SPIRIT

The righteous cry out, and the Lord hears them; he delivers them from all their troubles. The Lord is close to the broken-hearted and saves those who are crushed in spirit.

—*Psalms 34:17-18 NIV*

There is no better way to describe the feeling of trying to lose weight over and over again to no avail; it's like we're crushed in spirit. Maybe the first couple of times you tried you were able to write it off as something situational throwing you for a loop. Or maybe a vacation got in the way. But the 4th, 10th, and 24th time? Crushed in spirit.

David has such an amazing way with words. He is so honest with God and with himself. When he is in the depths of despair, he writes. He pours out his heart to

God. You can just tell he is on his knees with his face buried in his bed blankets. Or maybe he didn't even make it to the floor but instead just curled up in a little ball in his bed and vowed not to get up until God offered some sort of inspiration to pull him out of this abyss.

Thank God we have a way out! Thank God we have a reason to look up. Thank God we have assurance that we will be delivered from all our troubles. Thank God we have someone who will draw near to us in our absolute worst moments of doubt, fear, and defeat.

David has shown us that it is okay to be real. It is okay to fall down and stay there for a bit. It is okay to grieve a failure. But let's not stay there for too long. Jesus came to pull us out of despair by removing our sin from us. Jesus came to give us the ultimate gift of hope. I don't know how I would make it through without hope. Sometimes that is the only thing that gets us through.

> *And now, O Lord, for what do I wait? My hope is in you. Psalms 39:7 NIV*

In this verse, David doesn't even know what he is hoping for. He doesn't know what the outcome will be, but he decides to wait, knowing that his hope is in Someone who can do the impossible. And let me tell you—or maybe you want to tell me—"This struggle feels impossible." Put your hope in the One who IS hope.

Let's spend a few minutes giving God our troubles. Then spend the rest of the day placing our hope in Him. If a trouble comes to mind, give it to God and go back to hope.

21

THE LORD IS MY PORTION

Therefore, I have hope. Through the Lord's mercies we are not consumed, because His compassions fail not. They are new every morning; Great is your faithfulness. "The Lord is my portion," says my soul, "Therefore I hope in Him!" The Lord is good to those who wait for Him, to the soul who seeks Him.

—Lamentations 3:21-25 NKJV

The Lord is my portion. Now I know what you're thinking. *Really? Out of that whole set of verses, that is what you're going to focus on? You don't actually think that God is talking about our portion of food here do you?* No. No I don't.

What the Bible is saying here is that God will always be enough. But let's just say for one second that it was talking about food. Would it really be so crazy to pray for how much we eat and change the verse into our new mantra saying, "I will choose the Lord's portion"? God wants to be our sounding board. He wants to be involved in every area of our lives. Do you really think that God doesn't want to help you attain a healthier body? The Lord is good to those who wait for Him. If we pray to eat the Lord's portion before we eat and we wait for Him to help us, does it not make logical sense that God will help us eat HIS fill? I will hope in Him! I am seeking His help! And I know that on those days that I fall off the wagon, the Lord is right there waiting, with compassion, to help me back up with His mercies.

One of our problems is that we choose not to take him up on those new mercies immediately. We choose to believe we can only start over on the next day. Or we always have to start on a Monday. Or the first of the month. We cannot just choose to renew our efforts at the time we fall…can we? One of my favourite song lines is, "Maybe forgiveness is right where you fell… Salvation is here" (*Dare You to Move* by Switchfoot). I do not think the verse is being literal in saying that we can only get new mercies on a new day, in the morning. It is saying that the Lord is ALWAYS there to give you His new mercies. In your morning prayer, ask now and wait on the Lord. Forgiveness is right WHEN you fell…

not after a few hours or days worth of limping around. First, pray you won't fall. And then pray that if you do, you will get right back up with His mercies in tow and move on.

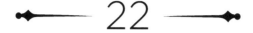

22

BE MERCIFUL

Be merciful, just as your Father is merciful.

—Luke 6:36 NIV

Mercy is compassion or forgiveness shown to someone who doesn't deserve it. Our Heavenly Father has shown great mercy to us. "While we were still sinners, Christ died for us" (Romans 5:8 NIV). Talk about mercy!

Our kids are constantly invoking situations where we need to be merciful. Our friends, spouses, and sometimes complete strangers require mercy from us. For some reason, the one person we tend to forget about being merciful to is ourselves.

There is a trendy movement right now of self-care and self-love. It is trying to help us learn to love ourselves. I'm not saying it is all bad. We do need to take care of ourselves and learn to accept ourselves as we are, but I think the trend is leaving out the God factor. As Christians, we are held to a higher and different standard than the world. We forget that the real self-love is actually God-love. When we put our focus on God instead of love of self, we enter into the plans He has for us. In other words, when we love God, we are doing our very best for ourselves. Instead of taking care of ourselves, we are filling up on God and giving ourselves over to Him to take care of us.

When we shift our mindset from self to God, that is an incredibly merciful act towards ourselves. God helps us to see His view of us. He shows us how treating our bodies according to His plan for us brings us freedom and peace. When we focus on self, all we can focus on are the restrictions, the failures, and the burdens. When we focus on God, His mercy pours over us and we remember why our lives can be full of grace and joy and freedom. Sometimes I do things like take a quiet bath so I can just pray and praise and be thankful. God has given me some of my best ideas and solutions in those times. Try to be more silent. Go for a walk with God instead of plunking in your ear buds.

23

CHRISTIAN MEDITATION

M editation is something that Christians tend to be wary about…and with good reason. The Christian way of meditation is much different from the world's version of it. The world sees meditation as trying to empty your mind. Christians know that God calls us to fill our minds with scripture and other pure thoughts. When we get really good at this, we can technically meditate all day long. It doesn't have to be a set time when you sit on your floor with a certain position of your hands. It doesn't have to include random noises.

Christian meditation is much more joyful. It is a constant state of prayer to our God all day long. It is singing a song of praise on your drive to work. It is picking a new verse to memorize every week. It is praying for our co-workers when we see them going through a hard time. It means showing grace to that one person who gets under your skin. Christian meditation is sitting down and reading your Bible. It is praying for the people on your prayer list. It is looking outside of yourself for answers to your hardest questions. It is looking to God. Always. It is getting in the habit of showing patience when all you want to do is lose it. It is being thankful, no matter the situation.

Keep this Book of the Law always on your lips;

Meditate on it day and night so that you may be careful to do everything written in it.

Then you will be prosperous and successful.

Have I not commanded you?

Be strong and courageous.

Do not be afraid; do not be discouraged, for the Lord your God will be with you wherever you go.

—Joshua 1:7-8 NIV

Start your meditation by finding a verse that inspires you to keep striving for your goals and start to memorize it. Health goals are just as attainable as any other goal. Anything and everything is possible if God wills it. Show Him you trust Him and His ways. Meditate on His words of encouragement. Meditate on the blessings He has given you. Renew your mind to Him daily and let Him protect your mind and be your stronghold against temptations. Let Him fill you with the joy of His salvation.

24

FOCUS ON THE UNSEEN

When I was trying to think of a good way to explain this concept, I thought of those pictures that really just look like a pattern. They used to have them in the Sunday newspaper that my dad would always get after church. Apparently if you stare at them just the right way you can see a picture in them. Now, I was one of those people who could never see them. Still can't. I tried to follow every piece of advice given to me: "Relax your eyes," "Look past it," "Look at just one spot and keep staring at it until it jumps out at you." When I couldn't see them, I'd hear, "How can you not see it? It's right there. I can't NOT see it."

This is an excellent interpretation of the difference between Christ-believers and non-believers. Think of the different language we use compared to non-believers. "I'll pray for you" vs. "I'll keep my fingers crossed for you." I'm sorry, but when has crossing your fingers for me ever actually done anything? I understand the intention is to support me, but as a Christian it means nothing. I know that crossing your fingers will have zero impact on my situation. I do know that the invisible act of prayer has a ton of power, and I trust that your prayers for me will have an impact in how the situation turns out.

"How can you be so calm when everything around you is falling apart?" Because I have faith that God's plan is the right plan.

"How can you be so thankful for your body when it isn't functioning or looking the way you want it to?" Because I'm still alive. And to live is Christ (Phil 1:21).

"How can you smile at the funeral of one of your most beloved family members?" Because I know they are walking through the gates of heaven towards an eternal life of joy and contentment.

"How can you live each moment with purpose even though it is so mundane?" Because God has given me purpose to choose to love Him and serve Him however I can…even if that means cleaning up after toddlers all day long. I will do it to the glory of God.

> *So, we are not giving up. How could we! Even though on the outside it often looks like things are falling apart on us, on the inside, where God is making new life, not a day goes by without his unfolding grace. These hard times are small*

potatoes compared to the coming good times;
the lavish celebration prepared for us. There's
far more here than meets the eye. The things we
see now are here today, gone tomorrow. But the
things we can't see now will last forever.

—2 Corinthians 4:16-18 The Message

Here's a silly story that brought great clarity for me back in high school when I had just broken up with a boyfriend. I like to think I can be a mind-over-matter person, so I came up with this plan. Whenever I would think of him, I decided to change to "singing" a song in my head. It was some church song. Every time I would think of him, I would sing it. Now some of you will scoff at the amateur solution, but try not to think of a pink elephant. Ha! Gotcha! You can't help it. Now try not to think of a chocolate bar. Gotcha again! You can't think of two things at once. Try to decide that at certain triggers you will think or sing something else. I found it to be a very effective coping mechanism. When I got over it, I found myself singing it more often just because. Find yourself a song and decide to sing it when a trigger shows up.

Your food and body issues of today will soon be forever overpowered by the unseen future we have in heaven. When we focus on the unseen ways of God, the day-to-day problems with food and exercise will start to take a back seat. If we change our thinking, God will change our mind.

25

NOURISHMENT

When it comes to brain-body nutrition, nourishment is part of a satisfying eating experience. It is also hard to measure how "nourished" we really are. It is not a number or a definition. It is not objective, it is subjective. It is a feeling. It is a natural response to a healthy eating experience. We feel nourished after we enjoy a meal. We feel nourished after eating when we can relax and fully appreciate what went into the meal we ate. We feel nourished when we take a deep breath after the meal and feel a sense of satisfaction. It is nearly impossible to feel this way if you are rushing through a meal or are completely distracted while eating. We are robbing ourselves of a sense of pleasure. This goes for a dessert as well. It is very hard to feel nourished by a piece of amazing birthday cake if we are internally punishing ourselves for eating it. Not only will we not truly enjoy it but the cravings for such food will probably not subside.

God created us to feel and enjoy pleasure. It is built into our DNA. It is built into our primary commandment as well: "Love the Lord your God with all your heart and with all your soul and with all your mind. This is the first and greatest commandment. And the second is like it: Love your neighbor as yourself" (Matthew 22:37-39 NIV). I think we can all agree that without love there is no such thing as pleasure. We were created to love, and we were created to enjoy that love. God, through Jesus Christ, has set us free from the burden of sin so we can fully enjoy all He has for us.

When it comes to nourishment, God tells us exactly what will nourish our bodies:

> *Trust in the Lord with all your heart and lean not on your own understanding; in all your ways submit to him, and he will make your paths straight. Do not be wise in your own eyes; fear the Lord and shun evil. This will bring health and nourishment to your bones.*
>
> *—Proverbs 3:5-8 NIV*

The most important element to take away from brain-body nutrition is to slow down. When we eat slower, our brain has a chance to process the pleasure we are experiencing. It is not an easy thing to do, but it really does change a lot in our body and brain processes. Try to extend meals at least five minutes today, working up to at least one half-hour meal a day if you can.

Trust the Lord.

Shun evil.

Love the Lord.

The recipe for nourishment is to fully revel in the Lord. The rest will follow.

26

OVERCOME SUFFERING WITH THANKSGIVING

I consider that our present sufferings are not worth comparing with the glory that will be revealed in us.

—*Romans 8:18 NIV*

God is not insensitive, but He is always truthful. The way we can read into that truth can sometimes appear harsh to us…at first. It can feel like He may be brushing off our hard times because He knows what is coming. It can feel like He just wants us to get over it when all we feel we can do is grieve something or someone. We can feel alone in our weight loss journey because we are embarrassed to tell anyone we failed again. But let us be certain: those are not truths. Would someone who loves you as much as the great I AM brush your problems aside?

Absolutely not. The devil, however, can shift our truths just slightly to make it appear that way.

What God is trying to show us is that the sufferings of this world will not last forever. He is offering us His perspective of the big picture. We cannot see the big picture. We cannot even fathom the big picture. What we can do, however, is give thanks. The Bible is constantly teaching us to look outside of ourselves and to be thankful for what we have. There is ALWAYS something to be thankful for. And really, we should not have to look far. Even if we cannot come up with anything "of this earth" we will ALWAYS have God to be thankful for.

Let them give thanks to the Lord for his unfailing love and His wonderful deeds for mankind, for He satisfies the thirsty and fills the hungry with good things.

—Psalms 107:8-9 NIV

Rejoice always, pray continually, give thanks in all circumstances; for this is God's will for you in Christ Jesus.

—1 Thessalonians 5:16-18 NIV

Look for God's perspective in your sufferings. Know that no matter how many times you fail, He will always be there. Know that He will always be there to step in when you finally reach the end of yourself. When you can finally admit that you cannot lose the weight yourself, God will answer immediately with something like, "I'm so glad you have realized that. Let me do it for you. Please just remember that you need to repeatedly renew your mind in congruency with My will. I will never leave you. I will never forsake you. If you will trust Me with this, I can show you the dreams I have dreamt for you. They will blow your mind and make your own dreams look like rubbish. I am holding you in the palm of my hand."

Today, let us trust God. Give your goals to God and thank Him for His overwhelming desire to be our number one fan.

27

WORRY OR PEACE?

Worry does not take away tomorrow's troubles. It takes away today's peace.

—Randy Armstrong

Worry is an ongoing struggle for so many people. Even as Christians we have our moments. It is something we continuously have to give over to God. Today I am going to let the words of an old hymn and Jesus himself wash over you and bring you peace. Meditate on these words and bask in the constant attention God pays to our smallest details.

He Loves Me Too!

God sees the little sparrow fall,
It meets His tender view;
If God so loves the little birds,
I know He loves me too.

He loves me too, He loves me too,
I know He loves me too;
Because He loves the little things,
I know He loves me too.

He paints the lily of the field,
Perfumes each lily bell;
If He so loves the little flow'rs,
I know He loves me well.

He loves me too, He loves me too,
I know He loves me too;
Because He loves the little things,
I know He loves me too.

God made the little birds and flow'rs,
And all things large and small;
He'll not forget His little ones,
I know He loves them all.

He loves me too, He loves me too,
I know He loves me too;
Because He loves the little things,
I know He loves me too.

by Maria Straub, 1874

Then Jesus said to his disciples: "Therefore I tell you, do not worry about your life, what you will eat; or about your body, what you will wear. For life is more than food, and the body more than clothes. Consider the ravens: They do not sow or reap; they have no storeroom or barn; yet God feeds them. And how much more valuable you are than birds! Who of you by worrying can add a single hour to your life? Since you cannot do this very little thing, why do you worry about the rest?

Consider how the wild flowers grow. They do not labor or spin. Yet I tell you, not even Solomon in all his splendor was dressed like one of these. If that is how God clothes the grass of the field, which is here today, and tomorrow is thrown into the fire, how much more will he clothe you—you of little faith! And do not set your heart on what you will eat or drink; do not worry about it. For the pagan world runs after all such things, and your Father knows that you need them. But seek his kingdom, and these things will be given to you as well.

Do not be afraid, little flock, for your Father has been pleased to give you the kingdom. Sell your possessions and give to the poor. Provide purses for yourselves that will not wear out, a treasure in heaven that will never fail, where no thief comes near and no moth destroys. For where your treasure is, there your heart will be also.

—Luke 12:22-34 NIV

28

WHAT IS TRULY VALUABLE?

For physical training is of some value, but godliness has value for all things, holding promise for both the present life and the life to come. This is a trustworthy saying that deserves full acceptance. That is why we labor and strive, because we have put our hope in the living God, who is the Savior of all people, and especially of those who believe.

—*1 Timothy 4:8-10 NIV*

I've been a fitness instructor since 2005. It was one of those things that just kind of fell in my lap. I decided I wanted to try and teach aquatic fitness because that seemed like the easiest one to teach. I took the course and it wasn't too bad. The funny thing was I was intimidated to try and teach it afterwards. I just figured it would be another thing that I just didn't end up following through on. God had other plans. Out of the blue I got a call asking me to teach. I have no idea how they got my contact information but that is how my journey into a hobby/career in fitness began. Soon after, I received an email from a local Pilates studio asking me if I wanted to train to teach with them. Again, I have no idea how they got my contact information but teaching Pilates had always been on my mind as it was one of my favourite exercises to do on my own.

This story could have been about any kind of push in a certain direction but mine happened to be about physical training. I can tell you that as someone who has been through some pretty low times, that physical training has brought me out of some major slumps. It got me to sleep during a time of insomnia. It brought my mood out of the gutter when I had tried everything else. It keeps me sane when my toddlers have…well, been toddlers.

When I look back on it, God instrumented a life full of fitness in order to draw me to Him. He used it to teach me that there is a time and a place for everything. I could teach pretty much any fitness class out there these days and the diversity brings me extreme relaxation. I am not a routine girl, and the fact that I could choose to run, do Pilates, lift weights, go to an aerobics class, or do some barre classes releases me from the stress that routine brings me. Yes, I realize that for most people routine brings peace, but it makes me feel choked. For a long time, I strived for routine and was successful at it for periods of time. God, however, always brought me back to His rhythm for me, which was variety. God used physical training to teach me how to live for Him. He used something with "some" value and turned it into something with eternal value. I learned ways to live my life to serve Him, and I encourage you to do the same. Find a tangible exercise that you enjoy and let God teach you something intangible that could save your life.

29

WHERE THE SPIRIT OF THE LORD IS, THERE IS FREEDOM

But whenever someone turns to the Lord, the veil is taken away. For the Lord is the Spirit, and wherever the Spirit of the Lord is, there is freedom. So, all of us who have had that veil removed can see and reflect the glory of the Lord. And the Lord—who is the Spirit—makes us more and more like him as we are changed into his glorious image.

—2 Corinthians 3:16-18 NLT

To put these verses into context I'm just going to give a very brief overview. Earlier in 2 Corinthians 3, Paul is explaining that we no longer live under the old covenant thanks to Christ. He is saying that we no longer need to cover our faces with a veil the way Moses did so the people would not see the glory of God on his face. Instead, now the veil covers the eyes of people who do not believe that Jesus Christ came to Earth to save them from their sins. That veil *covers their minds so they cannot understand the truth. And this veil can be removed only by believing in Christ (vs 14).*

BUT—and that is where our verse begins—when someone turns to the Lord, that veil is removed and we can accept the Spirit of God within us. When the Spirit comes to inhabit our souls, it brings freedom. Ah freedom. "It is for freedom that Christ has set us free" (Galatians 5:1). According to Paul, who wrote both of these verses, freedom is the reason for Christ. It is the reason why God sent His son to save the world. He went through all of that trouble to give us the best gift: freedom.

How many of us can honestly say that our current lifestyle brings freedom? Actually, let's narrow that down a little more because the reason you are reading this is to help you with your health and fitness goals. Do you feel that your health and fitness goals bring you freedom? I highly doubt it. It feels more like a stress. Like a burden. Like something that weighs on your mind the way not much else can. It is a daily struggle. A mental battle.

There's a good side and a bad side to this. I like to end on the good, so here is the bad first: this is not how it was meant to be. We were not meant to be burdened down so heavily by our choices. Interesting words, right? Choices? Yes, choices. I'm sure you feel that you don't have a choice in the matter. There are many reasons you chose your goals, one of which may be that a health professional recommended it. I get it.

The good news?

You still get a choice! You can choose to follow those "orders" with a frown or a smile. When you get orders like that, it means you have a chance to turn it around. Would they give you those orders if there was no hope? No. They would just put you in a bed and wait for the inevitable. We can take joy in the order. We can use it as incentive to encourage our efforts. We can also see it as a reason to continue to love the ones in our lives. Let's say a concerned family member brought up the topic. You may take it as an insult but, really, would anyone ever say anything to you if they didn't care? God is love first and foremost. God also brings freedom through Christ.

With that in mind, let's take this one step further and think of our goals as a free gift. Maybe even a freedom gift. We have the luxury to freely choose to take care of ourselves. Nobody can force us to do it. We are granted a free choice to make. God never forces anything on us. However, when we finally come around to His way of thinking, it feels like the easiest, most natural thing to do. It's like our choice was the final step to freedom. We didn't realize we needed to make a choice until it had already been made.

Now for the super good news. Just because life is hard doesn't mean you cannot feel free while living it. Have you ever gone through some kind of trauma or sin that has been weighing you down until you repented and healed? That freedom is tangible. It is tangible in a way that you never knew was possible until it was lifted from your shoulders. All of a sudden you can breathe freely. Your load has been lightened. Christ came to that specific part of your life and freed you from the burden. It is a miracle that only God can give. Give your health and fitness goals to Christ and allow Him to free you through your submission. Today, let's take time to praise God that we have the freedom to make choices that benefit us mentally, physically, and spiritually. This doesn't have to be a complicated prayer or process. Just talk to your Heavenly Dad. Have a conversation. Tell Him how you are feeling about this thought-changing process. Decide to trust Him in this. Then let it go.

30

WAIT FOR THE LORD

David went through every possible emotion as he wrote a good portion of the Psalms. Psalms 27 shows such confidence in our God. Even though evil advances and tries to surround us, still we will wait on the Lord. When the temptations of an unhealthy lifestyle suppress us, my heart says seek His face! I will wait for you. You are my ultimate helper! I will wait for Your way. You will always be there for me even when the people closest to me let me down. I will wait for You. Of whom shall I be afraid? No one. People are imperfect. God, You are forever. Teach me Your way, Lord, and I will be strong and wait for You. I will wait for You.

Spend today meditating on this passage.

> The Lord is my light and my salvation—whom shall I fear?

> The Lord is the stronghold of my life—of whom shall I be afraid?

When the wicked advance against me to devour me, it is my enemies and my foes who will stumble and fall.

Though an army besiege me, my heart will not fear; though war break out against me, even then I will be confident.

One thing I ask from the Lord, this only do I seek: that I may dwell in the house of the Lord all the days of my life, to gaze on the beauty of the Lord and to seek him in his temple.

For in the day of trouble he will keep me safe in his dwelling; he will hide me in the shelter of this sacred tent and set me high upon a rock.

Then my head will be exalted above the enemies who surround me; at his sacred tent I will sacrifice with shouts of joy; I will sing and make music to the Lord.

Hear my voice when I call, Lord; be merciful to me and answer me.

My heart says of you, "Seek his face!"

Your face, Lord, I will seek.

Do not hide your face from me, do not turn your servant away in anger; you have been my helper.

Do not reject me or forsake me, God my Savior.

Though my father and mother forsake me, the Lord will receive me.

Teach me your way, Lord; lead me in a straight path because of my oppressors.

Do not turn me over to the desire of my foes, for false witnesses rise up against me, spouting malicious accusations.

I remain confident of this: I will see the goodness of the Lord in the land of the living.

Wait for the Lord; be strong and take heart and wait for the Lord.

—Psalms 27 NIV

Find your favourite phrase from this passage and repeat it over and over in your head and out loud. Remember that scripture is the word of God and the devil shudders in fear when you stand strong with the sword of the spirit.

31

REJOICE IN SUFFERING

Dear friends, do not be surprised at the fiery ordeal that has come on you to test you, as though something strange were happening to you. But rejoice inasmuch as you participate in the sufferings of Christ, so that you may be overjoyed when his glory is revealed.

—*2 Peter 4:12-13 NIV*

Nothing brings us closer to Christ than our suffering. It tends to weaken us to a point where we end up on our knees. Our suffering makes our foundation in Christ that much stronger. It makes our joy that much more joyful.

I remember a time when I was doing pretty well in my life and a friend told me that she thought I was lucky to have gone through as much as I had. I thought that was an interesting way to put it, but I heard her out. She said that my faith has been tried and tested, and she could tell I had a strong relationship with God because of it. She said she hadn't ever had to go through that much, and she could see a difference between where we were at as Christians.

When I was thinking about it later, I realized that as much as the hard times were awful, I just couldn't regret them. I couldn't look back on them and say they were a worthless waste of my time because every time I had to go through something, I came out of it with an amazing lesson. My empathy grew, my understanding of grace exploded, and my judgment decreased.

I hope that as you go through this struggle, you are asking God what you are to learn from it. If nothing comes of it, it will have been a waste of your time. Maybe God is keeping you here until you get it. I am not saying that is the reason you are struggling, but it may be a part of it. Stop being a victim of your circumstances and start being proactive. Really get into it with God. Ask for direction. Ask for ideas of how to move forward. Ask for support. Try the following prayer, and then listen.

Dear Heavenly Father, thank you so much that You can work all things for Your good. Please show me the way You want me to go about getting healthy. Bring thoughts to my mind that will encourage me in the right direction. Help me to keep an open mind and heart as I listen for

Your response. If you see fit, please involve someone I trust in this process to offer advice and support. Please help me to keep my mind on You and to adopt the peace that can only come from You. In Jesus' name, Amen.

32

DELIGHT IN HIM

The Lord makes firm the steps of the one who delights in him; though he may stumble, he will not fall, for the Lord upholds him with his hand.

—Psalms 37:23-24 NIV

Today I want you to revel in the Lord and His promises. Pick a couple of verses from below to memorize and contemplate. What a blessing to be able to hear from the mouth of God whenever we want to through the Bible. Delight yourself in the Lord!

Consider it pure joy, my brothers and sisters, whenever you face trials of many kinds, because you know that the testing of your faith produces perseverance. Let perseverance finish its work so that you may be mature and complete, not lacking anything.

—James 1:2 NIV

Praise be to the God and Father of our Lord Jesus Christ! In his great mercy he has given us new birth into a living hope through the resurrection of Jesus Christ from the dead, and into an inheritance that can never perish, spoil or fade. This inheritance is kept in heaven for you, who through faith are shielded by God's power until the coming of the salvation that is ready to be revealed in the last time. In all this you greatly rejoice, though now for a little while you have to suffer grief in all kinds of trials. These have come so that the proven genuineness of your faith—of greater worth than gold, which perishes even though refined by fire—may result in praise, glory and honor when Jesus Christ is revealed. Though you have not seen him, you love him; and even though you do not see him now, you believe in him and are filled with an inexpressible and glorious joy, for you are receiving the end result of your faith, the salvation of your souls.

—1 Peter 1:3-9 NIV

Be joyful in hope, patient in affliction, faithful in prayer.

—Romans 12:12 NIV

Rejoice in the Lord always. I will say it again; Rejoice!

—Philippians 4:4 NIV

Until now you have not asked for anything in my name. Ask and you will receive, and your joy will be complete.

—John 16:24 NIV

For the kingdom of God is not a matter of eating and drinking, but of righteousness, peace and joy in the Holy Spirit.

—Romans 14:17 NIV

You make known to me the path of life; you will fill me with joy in your presence, with eternal pleasures at your right hand.

—Psalms 16:11 NIV

Use these verses as a meditation. Speak them over and over until God reveals to you the deep truth that will change your soul forever. All you must do is believe what you are reading and the Bible will come to life and change yours.

33

A SHIELD AROUND ME

God is the ultimate protector. Much of the Old Testament is filled with war, and God protects His people with a physical shield. He makes sure the right wars are won, even when His people are outnumbered. When Jesus came to Earth, God provided a tangible shield that created a bond and a base to which His people were able to learn from in person. When Jesus died, He provided the ultimate shield for our souls by conquering death and saving us from our sins. And when Jesus went back to heaven, God gave us the shield of the Holy Spirit, a constant friend and protector. Through Jesus and the Holy Spirit, we now have access to an army of angels that can protect and fight for us in the name of Jesus Christ.

As you go through this time of struggle and temptation, remember that your protection is just a word away. God always wants the best for us and is looking out for us no matter what, but He also loves when we get involved in our own security. He gives us unending blessings falling from heaven, so we just need to accept and use them to tip the war in our favour. It gives us a home court advantage when we, through Jesus, take control and use our prayers and protectors in our favour.

Even though this chapter of Psalms is about a physical war, it can be made to work for us as well. We know there is a spiritual opposition out there waiting for us to give up and fail again. We also know that God will always be a shield around us.

> *Lord, how many are my foes! How many rise up against me! Many are saying of me, "God will not deliver him."*
>
> *But you, Lord, are a shield around me, my glory, the One who lifts my head high. I call out to the Lord, and he answers me from his holy mountain.*
>
> *I lie down and sleep; I wake again, because the Lord sustains me. I will not fear though tens of thousands assail me on every side.*
>
> *Arise, Lord! Deliver me, my God! Strike all my enemies on the jaw; break the teeth of the wicked.*
>
> *From the Lord comes deliverance. May your blessing be on your people.*
>
> —*Psalms 3 NIV*

This is such a great prayer. Write this out and put it somewhere you can read it often. God will sustain and protect us always.

34

BEING PURPOSELY
CONSCIOUS

Our Father which art in heaven,

Hallowed be thy name.

*Thy kingdom come, Thy will be done in earth,
as it is in heaven.*

Give us this day our daily bread.

And forgive us our debts, as we forgive our debtors.

*And lead us not into temptation, but deliver us
from evil;*

*For thine is the kingdom, and the power, and the
glory, forever.*

Amen.

—Matthew 6:9-13 KJV

Thy kingdom come, Thy will be done in earth,
as it is in heaven.

The words of the Lord's Prayer are ones many of us grew up reciting. We could rattle them off without really knowing what we were saying. It was a prayer that, in a way, lost all meaning due to repetition. The funny thing is, we do that with so much of our lives and our Christian lives. We are unconsciously giving our lives to God. Now in some ways that sounds like a good thing— like it is so ingrained in us to go to God for everything that it's become second nature. In some cases, you're totally right. But in other instances, like the ones that we are really working on, really struggling with or really frustrated with the progress in, it's not enough.

When it comes to diet, exercise, and health, we tend to unconsciously give them to God. I've done it over and over again. Usually we start with good intentions. We pray about everything that goes into our mouths and for the motivation to workout. We put our faith in God that He will commit to our wants and needs without us truly committing them to Him in the first place. We throw up these relatively flippant, quick prayers that lack true dedication. Why do you think we do it? I think it's because most of us have tried over and over and OVER again to do this same thing. We've tried to lose weight. We've tried to eat healthier. And, like *The Lord's Prayer* when repeated many times, our prayers lose meaning because we don't really believe anything will actually change.

It is difficult to be purposefully conscious about things we have lost faith in. When we don't really believe what we are doing will work, it is difficult to commit.

God has taught me that when I become purposefully conscious it makes all the difference. Nutritionally, I am a firm believer in never cutting out any food or beverage. It starts a negative cycle that we never get out of. We restrict food → we crave that food → we binge on that food → we loathe ourselves for the weakness and lack of self-control → we restrict that same food.... Sound familiar?

Instead, God helped me truly commit to HIS will. His will might not take us to our ideal body. It might not make us a muscle model or a version of our body from 20/30/40/50 years ago. But it may just bring us to a place of health and wellness that helps us serve Him in a better way. Maybe it will make us more credible. Maybe it will help others take us seriously. Maybe it will bring us some self-esteem. God cares about our health…but not as much as He cares about our heart. He would rather have you commit your mind, body, and strength to His will than to your ideal body.

Thy kingdom come, Thy will be done, in earth as it is in heaven.

Try this prayer today:

God, please put Your kingdom right in front of me. I know You want me to be healthy so I may serve You better and longer. Let me see what Your will is and help me to do it. Help me to become purposefully conscious of Your will, even in the little things. Help me to see that I can trust You and that You have my best interest in mind. I pray that You take the desire for the unhealthy away and replace it with a desire for You. God, I know that anything, whether healthy or unhealthy, does me no good unless I KNOW You are more important. Being addicted to good things can be just as harmful to my spiritual life as to bad things. My thoughts should go to You more than anything else. Not your service, not spiritual warfare, not healing, but YOU. You are enough. Help me to know You better. To crave Your presence as much on Earth as I know I will in heaven. Amen.

35

NEITHER ICE CREAM NOR CHOCOLATE

For I am convinced that neither death nor life, neither angels nor demons, neither the present nor the future, nor any powers, neither height nor depth, nor anything else in all creation, will be able to separate us from the love of God that is Christ Jesus our Lord.

—Romans 8:38-39 NIV

When it comes to weight loss, money stress, physical diseases, or any kind of stress we are under, it always seems to try and take over our thoughts. Stress is the number one killer. It is the number one cause of any ailment in our bodies. It is the number one cause for our lack of peace. When we are stressed out there is no joy in life. We worry our minds in circles, getting worse and worse each time around.

There is also a stress cycle that happens with eating. We are frustrated with our eating habits so we decide to stop eating sugar, ice cream, or chips—whatever our treat of choice is. When we restrict the things we eat, we think about them constantly. If we finally cave and eat them, we feel terrible about ourselves and restrict all over again… only to give into the cravings.

Should we stop restricting what we eat? That's not the point.

The point is, we need to decide what we WANT to eat instead. If all we think about is the stuff we can't have, that's all we will want. If we are thinking about the food and drinks we can have, it changes our view on what we crave. Brain-body nutrition is complicated, but in the simplest form, it is changing how we think about food. For most people who have been in a cycle of dieting for a good portion of their lives, restricting foods is not the way to go about weight loss. I understand there is an ideal way to eat, but for many of us it is not realistic…especially when our emotions are caught up in it.

The bottom line is that no food choice we make will ever be able to separate us from God and His love for us. If angels or demons cannot separate us from the love of God, neither can a doughnut. Let's change our mindset to focus on that instead.

God loves you just the way you are. He will never love you more or less. He will love you through your successes and your failures just the same. Today, let's focus on the things we can control—like where our mind goes—and write them out. Let your mind dwell in the house of the Lord. Let it soak in the rays of peace. Let us give up our stressful ways and adopt the joy Christ has to offer. Working through problems is necessary. Dwelling on them is not.

36

GUARD YOUR HEART

Above all else, guard your heart, for everything you do flows from it.

—Proverbs 4:23 NIV

Your heart is the centre of who you are as a Christian. It's no accident that it is also the organ that keeps us alive. If your heart stops beating, the rest of your body dies. Heart disease is such a common problem these days. Maybe it is related, maybe not, but I certainly see the congruency as to how downtrodden we have become as Christians. We just don't care for our hearts enough; we are letting them get out of shape. If we do not exercise our hearts physically, how are they supposed to be strong and healthy? If we do not protect our hearts spiritually, we are much more prone to fall when attacks come. Heart attack anyone? Sorry. Dad joke.

Some of the best-known scriptures refer to our hearts. Let's take today to meditate on them. Let them sink in. Decide to memorize some or all of them. Our bodies (both spiritual and physical) are useless to us unless we take care of our hearts.

You will seek me and find me when you seek me with all your heart.

—Jeremiah 29:13 NIV

In their hearts, humans plan their course, but the Lord establishes their steps.

—Proverbs 16:9 NIV

Trust in the Lord with all your heart and lean not on your own understanding; in all your ways submit to him, and he will make your paths straight.

—Proverbs 3:5-6 NIV

Wait for the Lord; be strong and take heart and wait for the Lord.

—Psalms 27:14 NIV

Search me, God, and know my heart, test me and know my anxious thoughts.

—Psalms 139:23 NIV

Take delight in the Lord, and he will give you the desires of your heart.

—Psalms 37:4 NIV

Create in me a pure heart, O God, and renew a steadfast spirit within me.

—Psalms 51:10 NIV

For where your treasure is, there your heart will be also.

—Matthew 6:21 NIV

And the peace of God, which transcends all understanding, will guard your hearts and your minds in Christ Jesus.

—Philippians 4:7 NIV

Take my yoke upon you and learn from me, for I am gentle and humble in heart, and you will find rest for your souls.

—Matthew 11:29 NIV

37

FATHER KNOWS BEST

Therefore, I tell you, do not worry about your life, what you will eat or drink; or about your body, what you will wear. Is not life more than food, and the body more than clothes? Look at the birds of the air; they do not sow or reap or store away in barns, and yet your heavenly Father feeds them. Are you not much more valuable than they? Can any one of you by worrying add a single hour to your life?

And why do you worry about clothes? See how the flowers of the field grow. They do not labor or spin. Yet I tell you that not even Solomon in all his splendor was dressed like one of these. If that is how God clothes the grass of the field, which is here today and tomorrow is thrown into the fire, will he not much more clothe you—you of little faith? So do not worry, saying, "What shall we eat?" or "What shall we drink?" or "What shall we wear?" For the pagans run after all these things, and your heavenly Father knows that you need them. But seek first his kingdom and his righteousness, and all these things will be given you as well. Therefore, do not worry about tomorrow, for tomorrow will worry about itself. Each day has enough trouble of its own.

—Matthew 6:25-34 NIV

I love when Jesus is blunt but tactful. It makes me feel like He must be my Father. I was clearly made by Him because I have some of His blunt characteristics. Sometimes my delivery is less than optimal, but I am not perfect and I am still learning.

This passage is just so…parental. I just think of my three- and four-year-old kids asking "Why?" constantly. When I cannot come up with a good enough answer, I give the classic, "Because I said so." That should be enough. You, my children, should know by now that I am trying my best to do my best for you. Therefore, when you ask why you need to take a bath, and my "you stink" response doesn't sink in, I am just going to go with, "Because I said so!" We all know what a lack of bathing does but little kids do not. One day their "stinky peet" (feet) will not be adorable anymore.

I feel like Jesus is giving His children a very basic speech here so they can understand it as best as possible. Don't worry about what you eat or drink or wear. Worrying doesn't help anyone or anything. And then He basically repeats the same thing over again but in a different way. Maybe that way will sink in. But in the end, He just goes with, "Because I said so" by simply saying, "Do not worry."

God knows what you need and when you need it. Ask for His help and trust that He will come through for you in His perfect time. And when in doubt, just throw up your hands and surrender, knowing that Father knows best.

38

WORDLESS GROANS

In the same way, the Spirit helps us in our weakness. We do not know what we ought to pray for, but the Spirit himself intercedes for us through wordless groans.

—*Romans 8:26 NIV*

Thank goodness God takes our wordless groans as prayers! That must mean our tears, our head holding, our deep sighs full of stress, and our curling up in a little ball act as prayers too. Sometimes there are just no words. There are just overwhelming feelings of failure, frustration, self-hate, and sadness.

Just think about the time before Christ came to the Earth. You hear people wishing for the elaborate signs of those days, like having a donkey to converse with or a light of glory to pass by them. But I guarantee you that the people of those days would far prefer what we have now. We always have access to God. We don't need to spill blood to be forgiven. We speak our repentance and it is there. Having the Holy Spirit is the greatest gift we could ever hope for. Not only does He make God accessible all the time, but He forms words for us when we have none of our own. He speaks on our behalf and accepts the messages from God that appear in our heads and on our hearts.

He makes us feel that loving feeling; like a perfect dad holding his child in his lap. He assures us that our prayers are heard. He prompts us when to move and when to stay still. He urges us to forgive and release judgment. Ultimately, He brings us peace. We never have to question that our words fall on deaf ears. We can be assured that God takes them to heart and deals with them in his own way, in his own time.

The next time you are feeling low, think of the peace we have in us in the form of the Holy Spirit. Let that knowledge carry you to a place of thanksgiving and ultimately joy. Go back to one of your previous writing assignments and see if you can add to a list of things you can now be thankful for.

39

CONTENT WHATEVER THE CIRCUMSTANCES

I have learned to be content whatever the circumstances. I know what it is to be in need, and I know what it is to have plenty. I have learned the secret of being content in any and every situation, whether well-fed or hungry, whether living in plenty or in want. I can do all this through him who gives me strength.

—Philippians 4:11-13 NIV

Contentment
What a blessing to behold
To know trials and sorrows, yet still to be at peace
To know victory and accomplishment, yet
revel in the humility of Christ's sacrifice

To know sickness and death, and to be able
to sit by the rivers of tranquility
To know thanksgiving and success, yet be
washing the feet of the ones you love
To know anxiety and depression, yet letting your
face glow in the glory of the presence of God
To know rest and relaxation and still be
focused on our purposes for God
For every problem, there is encouragement
For every triumph, a meekness
In every situation, trust
Peace
Contentment

Choose to be content today. Choose to trust that God is in control today. Choose to make the sacrifice of Christ more important than the body He created for you to live in today. It is but temporary. God, alone, is forever.

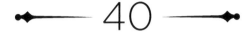

40

COME NEAR TO GOD

Submit yourselves, then, to God. Resist the devil, and he will flee from you. Come near to God and he will come near to you.

—James 4:7-8 NIV

Day forty. We made it. Let me tell you, this has been a journey for me. I hope you've had one too. If I'm being completely honest, I hope you have lost weight. But if I'm digging really deep, I hope you have grown closer to God. That is the only thing that is real in this life. The only thing worth striving for. The only reason why writing a book like this is of any worth.

Looking back over the highs and lows of this life, I can only be thankful for my journey. I can only be thankful that I hit rock bottom. I can only be thankful for my depression and other messy situations. And ultimately, I am coming around to being thankful that I gained my weight. If I had not, this book wouldn't have been written. I wouldn't have understood your struggle the way I do, and I wouldn't have cried as God's words came pouring out of me. God's purpose for my life is to keep on keeping on. It hasn't been to overcome, but to come out of it with lessons. With joy. With compassion, empathy, and a greater understanding of grace.

I hope that as you look back on your journey you do not feel that your purpose will start when you lose the weight. Your purpose is right now. Your purpose is to submit, learn, and love. God's main purpose for your life is to further His kingdom, so where you are right now is part of His plan. Look for it. Pray about it. Submit to the plan. Resist the devil and his foolish schemes. Come near to God. You will never regret it as He pulls you into His arms with more love than you can handle. That love will overflow into your life as peace and joy. If it took your weight to draw you nearer to God, it was worth it.

> *Therefore, we do not lose heart. Though outwardly we are wasting away, yet inwardly we are being renewed day by day. For our light and momentary troubles are achieving for us an eternal glory that far outweighs them all. So, we fix our eyes not on what is seen, but on what is unseen, since what is seen is temporary, but what is unseen is eternal.*
>
> *—2 Corinthians 4:16-18 NIV*

I encourage you at this moment to pray for everyone reading this book, or who will read it. Let's join together in encouragement and hope, knowing that *Gaining Christ* is the ultimate win.

WHAT NOW?

I wish I had some super wise advice for you on how to keep going. The truth is that I'm going through this with you. I am still trying daily to change my habits. I am quoting my verses when the triggers hit. I am still turning to God as I struggle with the weight. I will tell you what I keep telling myself:

> *Don't give up! Renew your mind daily. Read the Bible. Find the verses that come to life and dwell on them (I like the book of Romans in The Message—specifically Chapter 4). Pray constantly. Be thankful. Your mindset moves mountains—so focus on that. Submit to God. Trust God. Praise God.*

I plan to read this book over again. Every time I do, it brings tears to my eyes, which is what tells me these words were inspired by God, not myself. I would get sick of my own words. God's words have a pulse though. They come to life every time you read them.

Take care of yourself. Practice God-love on yourself, and let His mercy and grace transform you from the inside out.

When it comes down to it, I will tell you what I tell all of my clients: find what works for you. It may take time, but it is worth the search.

Thank you so much for sharing in this with me. I'll be praying for you as I hope you'll be praying for me.

Manufactured by Amazon.ca
Bolton, ON

17563525R00081